Ocular Applications of the Fugo Blade

Hampton Roy, M.D.
Associate Professor
Department of Ophthalmology
University of Arkansas for Medical Sciences
Little Rock, Arkansas

Daljit Singh, D.Sc.(Hon), M.S.
Professor Emeritus
Government Medical College, Amritsar, India
Baba Farid University of Medical Sciences
Faridkot, India
Director,
Daljit Singh Eye Hospital
Amritsar, India

Richard J. Fugo, M.D., Ph.D.
Professor
Department of Ophthalmology
Guru Nanak Dev University
Amritsar, India
Chief
Department of Ophthalmology
Mercy Suburban Hospital
Norristown, Pennsylvania

Wolters Kluwer | Lippincott Williams & Wilkins
Health
Philadelphia • Baltimore • New York • London
Buenos Aires • Hong Kong • Sydney • Tokyo

Senior Executive Editor: Jonathan W. Pine, Jr.
Senior Product Manager: Emilie Moyer
Senior Manufacturing Manager: Benjamin Rivera
Marketing Manager: Lisa Lawrence
Art Director: Doug Smock
Production Service: MPS Limited, A Macmillan Company

Printed in China

Library of Congress Cataloging-in-Publication Data

Ocular applications of the Fugo blade/F. Hampton Roy, Daljit Singh, and Richard J. Fugo, editors.
  p. ; cm.
Includes bibliographical references and index.
ISBN 978-1-60547-888-3 (hardback : alk. paper)
1. Eye—Surgery. 2. Electrosurgery. I. Roy, Frederick Hampton. II. Dalajita Singha, 1934- III. Fugo,
Richard J.
[DNLM: 1. Ophthalmologic Surgical Procedures—instrumentation. 2. Ophthalmologic Surgical
Procedures—methods. 3. Eye Diseases—surgery. 4. Eye Diseases—therapy. WW 168 O195 2010]
RE80.O38 2010
617.7'1—dc22

                                                                        2010011825

Care has been taken to confirm the accuracy of the information presented and to describe generally
accepted practices. However, the authors, editors, and publisher are not responsible for errors or omis-
sions or for any consequences from application of the information in this book and make no warranty,
expressed or implied, with respect to the currency, completeness, or accuracy of the contents of the publication. Application of the information in a particular situation remains the professional responsibility
of the practitioner.

The authors, editors, and publisher have exerted every effort to ensure that drug selection and dosage
set forth in this text are in accordance with current recommendations and practice at the time of publication. However, in view of ongoing research, changes in government regulations, and the constant flow
of information relating to drug therapy and drug reactions, the reader is urged to check the package insert
for each drug for any change in indications and dosage and for added warnings and precautions. This is
particularly important when the recommended agent is a new or infrequently employed drug.

Some drugs and medical devices presented in the publication have Food and Drug Administration
(FDA) clearance for limited use in restricted research settings. It is the responsibility of the health care
provider to ascertain the FDA status of each drug or device planned for use in their clinical practice.

To purchase additional copies of this book, call our customer service department at (800) 638-3030
or fax orders to (301) 223-2320. International customers should call (301) 223-2300.

Visit Lippincott Williams & Wilkins on the Internet: at LWW.com. Lippincott Williams & Wilkins
customer service representatives are available from 8:30 am to 6 pm, EST.

10 9 8 7 6 5 4 3 2 1

Dedication

This book is dedicated to the hard work and persistence of Dr. Daljit Singh, and to Dr. Richard Fugo, who developed the Fugo blade. Both men have spent countless hours developing and modifying this new technology.

–Hampton Roy

To my teacher, Prof. Man Singh Nirankari, F.R.C.S.

–Daljit Singh

Preface

The use of the Fugo blade is a new, evolving technology. Dr. Fugo is an ophthalmologist, and the technology has evolved faster in ophthalmology than in other fields.

Dr. Daljit Singh, an innovative ophthalmologist, has developed many of these procedures.

Conceptually, each chapter represents an anatomic area and details a disorder that is treated with the use of the Fugo blade. Clear photographs, illustrations, and text explain the approach to each surgical problem.

Acknowledgments

We would like to acknowledge the authors of each chapter. Each has done a splendid job of describing and illustrating his or her topic. We would also like to express our appreciation to Renee Tindall, author's editor; Dr. Paramjit Singh, anesthesiologist; Kanwar Mukesh, surgical assistant; Kamal Arora, media editor; and Surindar Singh, photo-artist.

Contributors

Amarjit Singh Atwal, MD
Director
Atwal Eye Care/Buffalo Eye Care Association
Medical Director/Founder
Buffalo Ambulatory Surgery Center
Buffalo, New York

Ephraim Singh Atwal, MD
Atwal Eye Care/Buffalo Eye Care Association
Buffalo Ambulatory Surgery Center
Buffalo, New York

Rakesh Bharti, MD
Consultant Dermatologist
Bharti Derma Care and Research Center
Amritsar, India

Harish K. Bisht, MD
Professor
Department of Ophthalmology
Sarojini Naidu Medical College
Agra, India

Vijeta Dhiman, MD
Resident
Department of Ophthalmology
Sarojini Naidu Medical College
Agra, India

C. Thomas Dow, MD
Associate Professor of Ophthalmology
University of Wisconsin
Madison, Wisconsin
Section Chief, Ophthalmology
Department of Surgery
Sacred Heart Hospital
Eau Claire, Wisconsin

Richard J. Fugo, M.D., Ph.D.
Professor
Department of Ophthalmology
Guru Nanak Dev University
Amritsar, India
Chief
Department of Ophthalmology
Mercy Suburban Hospital
Norristown, Pennsylvania

Taj Kirmani, FRCS Ed., FICS, FCPS
Professor of Opthalmology
Department of Opthalmology
Jinnah Postgraduate Medical Centre
Chief
Department of Opthalmology
Ziauddin Medical University
Karachi, Pakistan

Sunita Mohan, MD
Fellow VRS
Aditya Jyot Eye Hospital Pvt. Limited
Wadala, Mumbai, India

G. Russell Reiss, MD
Staff Cardiothoracic Surgeon
Division of Cardiothoracic Surgery
George E. Whalen VA Medical Center
Salt Lake City, Utah

Saran K. Satsangi, MBBS, MS
Professor
Department of Opthalmology
Sarojini Naidu Medical College
Sarojini Naidu Eye Hospital
Agra, Uttar Pradesh, India

Amrik Singh, FRCS
Professor of ENT
Guru Ram Das Medical College
Amritsar, India

Daljit Singh, D.Sc.(Hon), M.S.
Professor Emeritus
Government Medical College, Amritsar, India
Baba Farid University of Medical Sciences
Faridkot, India
Director,
Daljit Singh Eye Hospital
Amritsar, India

Indu R. Singh, MS
Consultant Ophthalmologist
Dr. Daljit Singh Eye Hospital
Amritsar, India

Kiranjit Singh, MS
Consultant Ophthalmologist
Dr. Daljit Singh Eye Hospital
Amritsar, India

Ravijit Singh, MS
Consultant Ophthalmologist
Dr. Daljit Singh Eye Hospital
Amritsar, India

Seema K. Singh, MS
Consultant Ophthalmologist
Dr. Daljit Singh Eye Hospital
Amritsar, India

Arun Verma, MD
Opthalmologist
Senior Consultant
Department of Opthalmology
Dr. Daljit Singh Eye Hospital
Amritsar, India

Contents

SECTION III: NONOPHTHALMIC APPLICATIONS OF THE FUGO BLADE 169

Section I
Introduction to the Fugo Blade

The Origins of the Fugo Blade RICHARD J. FUGO

After receiving my PhD in neurophysiology and biophysics, I pursued my medical degree in ophthalmology at Hahnemann University in Philadelphia. Upon graduating in 1979, I started my private practice in my hometown. The practice grew quickly, but nonetheless, I found I had a great deal of spare time at my disposal. I decided to take advantage of the free time to hone my surgical skills, and I began to perform a great deal of eye surgery on animals. As I did so, I became very disenchanted with the capabilities of the cutting instruments I was using.

I began practicing with many different devices, including electrosurgical devices, diamond blades, sapphire blades, and scalpels. The shortcomings of each device led me to realize that we really did not have a good surgical device. My background in electrophysiology and biophysics led me back again and again to electrosurgery. I tested many different electrosurgical units, most of which I was borrowing from the hospital where I was working. I found that all of the units worked poorly. They all burnt the tissue and the surgical area, giving off fumes that smelled disturbingly like burning human flesh.

I read every article that I could on electrosurgery and even visited with experts in the field of electrosurgery. I spent a great deal of time trying to understand how electromagnetic radiation functions in making an incision. Textbooks provided superficial explanations, so I consulted advanced physics descriptions written by eminent physicists. I found a great deal of divergence among these experts in their opinions on electromagnetic fields and their interaction with matter.

Eventually, my extensive study of the field of electrosurgery and electromagnetic field interaction with matter brought me to a rather interesting conclusion. I formed the opinion that our concept of the electromagnetic field as proposed in textbooks and by most authors in electrical engineering and physics is incorrect. I buried myself in advanced physics and electrical engineering texts and attempted to integrate theories of optics with those of electrical engineering. I soon realized that we had a gross misunderstanding of the "photon." If my own theory regarding the photon was correct, then electrosurgical systems were designed incorrectly. I made up my mind to design a new, high-efficiency electrosurgical system based on my new concepts of the interaction of electromagnetic waves and matter.

The key ingredient to my paradigm-changing electrosurgical system was a highly efficient absorption of electromagnetic waves by matter. My intense studies of advanced physics were rocky and stormy, but were filled with moments of enlightenment. I came to realize that space was not a void, but rather was filled with energy in the form of electromagnetic and gravitational waves. Electric fields and magnetic fields are not separable; instead, they are differing perceptions of the same entity, namely an electromagnetic field. Electromagnetic fields are actually composed of Planck electromagnetic quanta that ophthalmologists call "photons." All matter is constantly emitting and absorbing electromagnetic fields in order to maintain an energy balance in the molecular lattice of the universe. Matter and electromagnetic fields are different forms of energy existing in interfaced or overlapping dimensions. The speed of light is a characteristic of the dimension in which electromagnetic radiation exists rather than a true speed. This is how electromagnetic fields instantaneously upon inception travel at the speed of light, whereas matter cannot travel at the speed of light even when propelled by immense energy levels. Therefore, matter is a character of the "slow" dimension, whereas electromagnetic fields are a character of the "fast" dimension.

This is, of course, a simplification, since slow and fast are relative terms and a true relativistic discussion of this is warranted. Nonetheless, my aim is to present just a few of the thoughts that were the basis for my approach to electrosurgery. If you think about it, it makes a lot of sense. The object of electromagnetic surgery is transferring electromagnetic energy into matter and using this energy to create an incision in matter. Because the objective of the electrosurgical systems has been to pass sufficient energy through matter to create heat—effectively causing a burn in matter—they have classically been extremely inefficient. I objected to the caustic nature of the burn and was sure that there must be a way to elevate the bond energy of the molecular lattice without creating oxidation, charring, or burning in the path of the incision. This ambitious goal led me and my colleagues to many failures along the way.

Our Fugo blade project encountered immense hurdles, yet a door would always open at the 11th hour to allow us to pass through. After about 10 years of work, we found that system power was not actually the most important aspect of an electrosurgical system. Instead, an energy source had to be tuned such that it had a high-efficiency component to transfer the energy into a molecular bond lattice. So as we tuned our system to transfer energy in an efficient manner, the amount of total system energy required actually decreased. (For this reason, the device that is currently used for capsulotomy, glaucoma, and iridotomy is powered by rechargeable flashlight batteries. The device is sharper than a diamond blade and can cut for over an hour, yielding incision walls that are pristine, as demonstrated by histologic studies from major medical centers across the United States.

Word of our progress got out, and in 1997 I was invited to lecture at the American College of Eye Surgeons. It was there that I met Dr. Daljit Singh. Dr. Singh clearly understood how technology works and instinctively knew that this was the device that he had been waiting for to revolutionize his surgical capability. He believed that it was a "great equalizer" that would provide the same quality of care to all in both industrialized and third world nations. Our united goal to bring about universal health care paved the way for a very close friendship that has spanned years and oceans.

Since our first meeting, Dr. Singh has followed through on his promise to stand by and work with me on the Fugo Blade Project. He is still actively involved in the project on a humanitarian level. The Dr. Daljit Singh Eye Hospital in North India is modern, clean, efficient, and extremely well equipped. At his hospital, Dr. Singh has completed more clinical studies over the course of 10 years than anyone else in the world and is truly *the* expert on clinical applications of Fugo blade technology.

The Fugo Blade Project has truly taken on a life of its own by receiving outstanding approvals both nationally and internationally. The U.S. Food and Drug Administration has cleared the device for use in capsulotomy, a novel form of glaucoma surgery called "transciliary filtration" or "Singh filtration," iridotomy, and dental surgery. Protocols also currently exist within and outside the field of ophthalmology. We are developing fantastic systems that have immense potential to radically change the way that surgeons perform all types of surgery. The device will give the surgeon high-efficiency incisions that have pristine incision walls that achieve hemostasis without charring or burning, yet still provide resistance-free cutting. This technology also decontaminates incisions; plasma is the key. We are now working on novel techniques that will provide surgical fields with prolonged antimicrobial characteristics and with accelerated healing capabilities. Plasma ablation of bone is also a fascinating field that has unlimited potential.

One point repeatedly raised by doctors who have used our plasma cutter is that the Fugo blade allows them to do things that are impossible without this device. This is absolutely true. We believe the Fugo blade is the first paradigm-shifting technology since the introduction of the laser back in the mid-20th century. Thus, it allows us to approach previously impossible tasks in a straightforward and surgeon-friendly fashion. The Fugo blade takes us into uncharted territories to dramatically improve the delivery of desperately needed health care to patients worldwide. We believe that the Fugo blade offers the greatest hope for delivering health care in a more efficient and effective manner to all races, religions, and economic classes.

The future of the Fugo blade is great and offers unlimited avenues to dramatically improve the entire field of surgery.

The Biophysics and Mode of Operation of Plasma Surgery

RICHARD J. FUGO and
DALJIT SINGH

Science is a sand castle. It is beautiful, but the deeper
we dig, the less formidable is the foundation.

— Daljit Singh

In this chapter we share the experiences that drew us to harnessing plasma energy in the program that we refer to as "Fugo blade technology." Much of what has come to surprise us is not based on what is known in the scientific community, but rather on what is unknown, unclear, or just incorrect. The plasma technology of the Fugo blade has prompted us to continuously revise our ideas about the intricacies of physics. The more we persevered along the path toward understanding the heartbeat and pulse of plasma, the more we found that the foundation of academic physics was filled with contradictions and inaccuracies.

We will attempt to explain the science behind plasma surgery in a straightforward, physician-friendly manner, eliminating math and physics jargon as much as possible. Rather than teaching mathematics, it is our hope that this text will allow the reader to understand and mentally visualize the subject matter. Our goal is to create a clear, correct view of physics while developing in the reader an understanding of the basic concepts of this field. When topics found in basic physics books are not correct, we will tell you this. When you read advanced physics, you will realize that much of the material found in a first-year physics book are "guesses" or "educational crutches," but is not actually correct. We will point out these inaccuracies in order to provide a firm understanding of the topic at hand.

Plasma

Types of Matter

The universe is composed of four states of matter: solids, liquids, gases, and plasmas. Although 99% of the universe is composed of plasma, it is the least understood state of matter simply because the other three states are those predominantly found on Earth. Our planet is one of the rare cases in the universe, a form of oasis containing a preponderance of non-plasma matter. (Note that the plasma state of matter must not be confused with blood plasma.) Plasma itself is highly protean, since more forms of plasma exist than do different forms of the other three non-plasma states of matter combined.

All four states of matter are combinations of atomic particles and energy fields, including electromagnetic (EM), atomic bond, and gravitational, among others. Solids, liquids, and gases (also called "SLG matter") contain atomic structures—electrons, protons, and neutrons. Neutrons (neutral charge) and protons (positive charge) are contained in the nucleus of the atom and are held together by nuclear atomic bond fields. Electrons are negatively charged particles that orbit around the nuclear particles in specific orbits held in place by various field energies. Structurally, an atom is often depicted in basic texts as a miniature solar system with a sun (the nucleus containing the protons and neutrons) and elliptically circling planets (the electrons).

Our miniature solar system view of the atom makes things look neat and clean, but it simply is not so. The reason is that we really do not understand the fundamentals of the atom. For example, we cannot explain the inner structure or "micro-anatomy" of electrons, protons, or neutrons. Physicists have attempted to explain these basic concepts by giving us "definitions," but they really do not understand these structures. Another point of contention is that texts show the orbits of various electron levels as specifically shaped configurations beginning with a simple circular or elliptical orbit that can greatly increase in orbit complexity. The trouble is that these proposed orbits are not really taken seriously except in providing a simplistic explanation. So we actually do not understand the structure or the dynamics of an atom. In addition, an accelerated charged particle—e.g., an electron—moving around a nucleus should cause an EM wave to be emitted by the electron. That is the basic mechanism of a radio transmitter. The production of this EM field would require the electron to expend energy at such a rate that it would crash into the nucleus in less than one millionth of a second. In this case, the atom would be, in effect, a "miniature" radio transmitter. However, electrons traveling in their atomic paths do not emit an EM field and they do not crash into the nucleus. Although we could give you possible reasons, we do not understand why these things happen in the manner in which they do.

Early Physics: Delving Deeper into the Structure of the Universe

In the late 1800s and early 1900s, we believed that the universe was filled with a substance called "ether," which in turn bathed all the particles and energy. Then, around the time of Einstein, the scientific community came to believe that the ever-present ether did not exist, but rather that the universe was largely a vacuum surrounding the atoms and atomic particles. Over the past 20 years, many advanced physicists have become convinced that the original ether idea was actually correct.

The question that remains is "What exactly composes ether?" Many believe that it may be composed of energy fields such as EM and gravitational waves. For example, if you turn on your television to a blank channel, you can see a picture of "snowy" background noise. Though not much thought was given to background noise on the TV, it was found during the mid-1900s that this snowy picture was actually generated

by EM radiation originating from the Big Bang creation of the universe. This EM field is everywhere, and it may well be part of the universe's ether. In that vein, *Scientific American* once created a series of images of the universe using several different cameras, each imaging different wavelengths of the EM field. These images vividly showed great variation in how the universe is perceived, depending upon the capability of the imaging device. Thus, what we humans see is a far from complete reality; for example, we have no way of visualizing "dark matter," which composes a large part of our universe.

All four states of matter are a mixture of atomic particles and field energy, including EM fields, short-range nuclear attractive forces for nuclear particles, coulomb repulsive forces for nuclear particles, gravitational forces, and so on. In general, solids, liquids, and gases possess much lower energy levels than plasma does. Atomic fusion occurs inside stars, wherein nuclei beginning with hydrogen (the smallest atom) are forced or fused together to create larger atoms. This process of fusion repeats itself until all the atoms in the periodic table are created. These atoms are then discharged by the star and expelled into space. So, all the atoms that comprise our earth were at one time manufactured in the belly of a star and were in the plasma state.

Plasma is the state of matter that generally possesses the highest level of energy. Also, more forms of plasma exist than all of the other types of matter combined. It is just that Earth contains mostly low-energy forms of matter, such as solids, liquids, and gases, which is why we are unfamiliar with the plethora of plasma forms. Plasma is often described as "a sea of protons in an ocean of electrons," wherein these charged particles gracefully oscillate to and fro within energy fields to make up the heart of plasma. Thus, Earth is an oasis of low-energy matter sitting in a universe composed largely of high-energy plasma. In basic terms, plasma is a mixture or a "soup" of electrons and protons in an intense energy field, mostly an EM field.

As the energy level of an atomic structure increases, the bond energy is overcome and electrons are discharged into space. In this manner, SLG matter is once again recycled back into the plasma state. As more energy is being absorbed by the atomic structure, more free electrons are being discharged from the atomic lattice. Some of the parameters used to describe various forms of plasma include electron density, electron kinetic energy, and the frequency of the plasma electrons. The protons and electrons swing rhythmically back and forth in the intense EM field. Recall that Einstein taught us—with his famous "$E=MC^2$"—that all particles and fields are forms of energy. Thus, atomic components are constantly reacting with fields. Recall that as charged particles accelerate, they emit EM fields into space, while these same particles are simultaneously absorbing other field energy—e.g., photon absorption by matter. This is the basis of photosynthesis, sight, suntan, and so on. Therefore, atomic particles are constantly recycling surrounding EM fields by simultaneously emitting EM fields and absorbing other EM fields.

Thus, we can see a constant dynamic interaction and exchange of energy from fields by the molecular lattice that composes solids, liquids, and gases—namely, constantly absorbing EM energy fields while simultaneously emitting EM energy. The absorption and emission of energy is truly dynamic. Does every atomic particle absorb every EM field that comes near it, like a miniature vacuum cleaner? No it doesn't. As people have preferences for certain foods, atoms have preferences for certain EM fields. We do not visually perceive everything around us because human photoreceptors have an affinity for specific EM fields, i.e., photons. Recall how the focused EM field of a yttrium:aluminum:garnet (or YAG) laser reacts differently with the irises of different patients. If matter is sensitive to a specific EM field energy, it absorbs it like a sponge does water. However, as the atom becomes progressively less compatible with or sensitive to a given EM field, it will progressively absorb the field less effectively. It is much like a radio. If a radio is tuned to a specific frequency, it will effectively absorb the EM field (radio wave), whereas increasing the distance of the frequency of the radio's tuner mechanism from a given EM frequency, decreases the efficiency of absorption, and we will hear progressively more static. We emphasize that this principle is one of the basic tenets upon which Fugo blade technology is based. As we condition the output signal (i.e., the EM field) of the Fugo blade such that it is highly absorbed by the molecules in the intended field of incision, we produce a highly efficient interaction between molecules and EM fields that generates a unique, controlled form of plasma.[1]

Since plasma is an EM field embedded with oscillating electrons and protons, it reacts much like radio waves react with a radio tuner. If we condition our plasma to be compatible with a specific matter, then that matter will absorb the EM field of the plasma in a highly efficient manner. As matter absorbs progressively more energy, the bond energy of the molecular lattice is superseded, wherein the large molecule shatters into small pieces, much like shattering a glass pane on a concrete floor. As an incision is made using the Fugo plasma technology, molecular fragments stay in the plasma cloud for only a fraction of a second, where they serve as the fuel for the plasma cloud and are then discharged out of it. This process is similar to those atoms that have undergone fusion in a star, as described earlier in this chapter, and are then ejected from the star into space. Because the material in the path of the intended incision is the actual fuel for the Fugo blade plasma, Fugo blade technology creates "primary plasma."[2] Older, less efficient plasma cutters used fuels such as argon or butane to generate plasma. The kinetic energy generated from this form of plasma cloud was then used to "burn" a path through matter, which is why these systems operate on "secondary plasmas." These secondary plasma systems are outdated, inefficient, and caustic to tissue.

Dimension Theory of Matter and Energy Fields

We should provide a short discussion to describe some very important characteristics regarding atomic particles and energy fields. Let us begin by addressing the doubt that exists among influential physicists regarding the concept of relativity as has been taught by Albert Einstein. First, we must appreciate that the concepts of "fast" and slow" are not simple, since it depends on the position of the observer. Relativity states that nothing can move faster than light (a small region of the EM spectrum), yet numerous books have been written about movement at "superluminal" speeds, faster than the speed of light. It is quite subjective and relativistic to define human movement as "slow" while dubbing light as "fast." If you were a miniature observer sitting on a single photon traveling across the sky, then the photon upon which you are riding would appear to move slowly while the Earth below you would appear to move very fast, at the speed of light. As an observer on Earth, we see the motions and dynamics of all forms of atomic particles to be slow in comparison to those of EM fields. For example, the speed of a jet fighter is considered to be relatively slow in comparison to that of light, a form of EM field with a frequency of 10^{14} cycles per second and a moving velocity of about 299,792.5 km per second. The velocity of light keeps being revised and updated, since we still do not know its precise value. How could it be that we have been unable to exactly measure the speed of light? We know that light can react with the matter near it, but its actual velocity has eluded us. Photons can also be deflected by gravity; therefore, light rays moving past the sun will have their paths "bent." Because of this, stars are often referred to as "gravitational lenses," since they bend or diffract light. Before we can hope to understand physics, it is imperative that we understand the concepts of slow and fast. Einstein's theory of relativity highlighted the significance of these concepts, which at first appear simple and an issue of common sense. We must keep in perspective that EM fields comprise the atmosphere through which charged atomic particles move while constantly and simultaneously absorbing and emitting various EM fields. Thus, the flow of energy in the universe is constantly being recycled.

Many physicists believe that our universe contains multiple overlapping planes of existence, or dimensions, that allow certain interactions between the dimensions while retaining their own distinct dimensional characteristics of existence. Therefore, could it be that matter and EM radiation exist in different dimensions? If this were the case, then this would certainly explain much of the confusion in our attempt to quantitate and explain EM radiation and matter. In this scenario, the velocity of light would not be an actual speed of movement or velocity in our dimension, rather it would be a description of existence for the dimension in which light actually exists. This would help to explain why the concepts of light and relativity presented in books, do not often make sense. As an example, you can flip on a light switch, which allows the filament of the bulb to give off light, for which each and every photon moves at the speed of light from its very moment of conception. They do not begin at zero speed and rapidly accelerate to the speed of light; rather, they always and only exist at the speed of light because this is the nature of the dimension in which they exist. Articles that report "slowing down the speed of light" are not reporting what occurs to the speed of a given photon.[2] As light travels through space, photons can be absorbed by matter. While absorbed, the photon is no longer moving as an EM field, but rather it exists as energized matter. Therefore, the overall voyage of a photon being converted to energized matter and then re-emerging as a photon will cause a ray of light to appear to have slowed down because of its existence in the energized matter state. In this way, the overall velocity of the light is slowed down, whereas the velocity of a photon is not.

Furthermore, if we attempt to accelerate solid matter—e.g. an electron—to the speed of light, it would take a gigantic amount of energy. Governments and universities have built particle accelerators that are bigger than a football field and require immense energy, yet they have still been unable to achieve this goal. Yet, turn on the light and each photon that it emits moves at the speed of light from its very inception. How is it that we cannot make an electron travel at the speed of light and yet photons always traveling at the speed of light are unable to be slowed down? Clearly, using speed or velocity to measure the differences of objects in different dimensions is merely a rough, inaccurate method of description. Understanding this issue allows us to have a more precise understanding of the components of plasma—namely, the EM field and the matter.

This existence of visible light, a small part of the EM spectrum existing in a separate dimension and governed by its own principles, is the reason for the paradox of light appearing simultaneously as a wave form and as small particles referred to as "photons." The waveform-versus-particle debate has been argued extensively in the literature, with little clarity being shed on the topic. The frequency spectrum of the EM field is massively huge, definable only by high-order exponents, whereas visible light accounts for only a minute section of the EM spectrum. In the early 1900s, scientists defined the energy content of each frequency of the EM spectrum with the formula:

$$E = h V,$$

where E is the energy of the photon, h is the universal constant known as Planck's constant, and V is the frequency of the photon.

Since the spectrum of frequencies of the EM field is almost limitless, there appear to be limitless types of protons as well. This has been confusing to some because nature usually functions on simple mechanisms. Recall that the nucleus has two basic particles—protons and neutrons. So, how is it that the types of photons in the entire EM spectrum account for nearly limitless types of photons? One interesting possible explanation is based on the types of waveforms—namely, transverse waves and longitudinal waves. Classic physics of the 1900s postulated that EM fields are transverse waves whereas sound waves are described as a longitudinal wave. Transverse waves oscillate repeatedly upward then downward, like waves on the top of the ocean. On the other hand, longitudinal waves are repeating zones of highly dense, compressed particles followed by zones of low-density, rarified particles. Sound waves are longitudinal waves with repeating zones of compressed air molecules followed by rarified air molecules. If we were to postulate that light is a longitudinal waveform rather than a transverse wave, then it would be possible to use a single type of photon to account for every frequency in the entire EM spectrum. This single photon type certainly complies with nature's rule of simplicity. High frequencies would result in a short pulse of dense photons hitting matter, which raises the energy level of the molecular lattice. This would be followed by an equally short pulse of low-density photons hitting matter, providing less energy dissipation by the molecular lattice before it is hit by another high-density wave of photons that further raises the energy level of the matter. Slower frequencies would possess longer zones of high-density photons followed by equally long zones of low-density photons, which would allow the matter to more effectively dissipate accumulated energy. All this could be accomplished by a single type of photon and would eliminate the paradox of EM wave versus EM particle as seen in the transverse EM wave model.

We want to underscore that we did not expend effort and time describing the EM field as a mere academic exercise. You cannot understand or appreciate plasma unless you firmly grasp the concept of the EM field. The EM field is the backbone and skeleton of all plasma.

As stated earlier, plasma has many more forms and configurations than all the other three states of matter combined. One of the beautiful aspects of plasma is that you can condition and modify it, providing an almost limitless array of plasma forms. Early in our research, we filmed a plasma cloud that had a discrete periodicity, which we were able to modify and morph into a spectrum of organized structures. One of these images contained periodic nodes and looked like a barber's pole, prompting us to name the image the "barber pole photo" (Figs. 2.1 and 2.2).

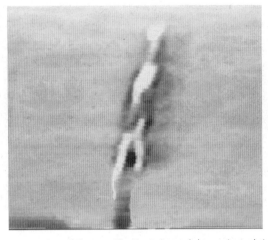

Figure 2.2. High-magnification view of the activated tip presented in Figure 2.1, right. We see the precise periodic nature of the plasma. This is changed by minimally altering the tuning parameters of the Fugo blade console.

The Fugo Blade in Plasma Surgery

The Fugo blade is a solid-state electronic system that produces efficient plasma surgery with primary plasma. The technology is protected by over 100 patents worldwide. The system has been cleared by the U.S. Food and Drug Administration (FDA) for human applications including:

anterior capsulotomy for cataract surgery,

glaucoma filtration from the posterior chamber of the eye through the pars plicata,

iridotomy for glaucoma, anterior chamber or intraocular lenses (IOLS) and implantable contact lenses (ICLs), and

dentistry.

The Fugo blade is portable and easily operates on batteries or wall current (Fig. 2.3). The system is a complete solid-state electronic system powered by low levels of electrical energy. The system emits a conditioned EM wave.[3] In a sense, it is an EM wave transmitter that transmits a specially conditioned EM wave that has quite unique characteristics. This EM wave is conditioned such that it is highly absorbed by the matter in the intended path of incision. EM energy may be reflected by matter, pass through matter, or be absorbed by matter. Recall that visible light may reflect from the surface of a mirror, x-rays can pass through a hand, and visible light is absorbed by photoreceptors. By making the transmitted EM field of the

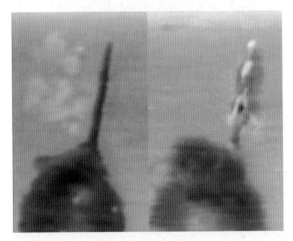

Figure 2.1. High-speed filtered imaging of Fugo blade cutting filament. **Left:** Inactivated cutting filament is polelike and lacks plasma; therefore, it has a dark color. **Right:** Activated Fugo blade cutting filament is precisely tuned such that the plasma presents a periodic pattern, which was coined "barber pole plasma" because it resembles a barber pole.

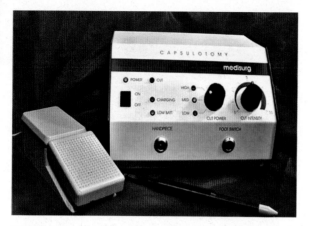

Figure 2.3. The Fugo blade system includes a battery-powered electronic console, an activation foot pedal, an ergonomic hand piece, and a charging unit (not shown).

Fugo blade resonant with the matter in the intended path of incision, we create a device that allows matter to literally suck the transmitted EM field into the molecular lattice of the intended incision path. This highly efficient absorption of the EM field by matter reduces the total amount of energy needed to perform its functions. This is why the Fugo blade works equally well on batteries or wall current. Although the Fugo blade looks like a standard electrosurgical system, its mode of action is that of a laser. The Fugo blade requires no grounding plate, and the cutting tip is blunt when it is inactive. When activated, this blunt cutting tip cuts more sharply than a diamond blade. The blunt cutting filament is a transmitting antenna in the truest sense. This ability to focus, concentrate, and control a transmitted EM field is a very powerful capability. This is one of the hallmark capabilities of Fugo blade technology.[4]

Let us give a simple example to demonstrate just how powerful it is to possess the capability of concentrating and focusing energy. If we captured the electrons that light one 100-W light bulb for just 1 second in a magic bottle, and then collected an identical set of electrons in a second magic bottle, we would then be able to measure the repulsive force of the two bottles filled with negatively charged electrons as we moved the bottles closer together. At 1 yd of separation between the two bottles, they would possess an enormous repulsive force, capable of lifting ten average-sized battleships out of the water simultaneously. Just think that such power comes from collecting and controlling the energy from a single 100-W light bulb that was lit for two 1-second periods. This is precisely why the focused EM field of the Fugo plasma blade is so powerful. The absorption of this focused EM field into the molecular lattice has immense ability to alter and

rearrange the structure of a molecular lattice in an intended field of incision.

We will now explain the difference in action between a standard electrosurgical system, a laser, and the Fugo blade. The mode of action of standard diathermy is demonstrated in Figure 2.4. Recall that

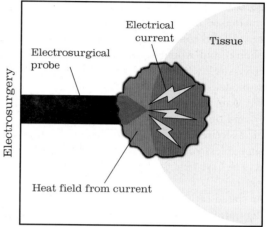

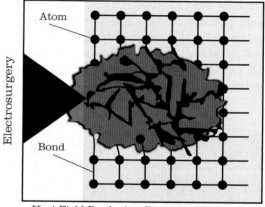

Figure 2.4. A diagram of standard electrosurgery.
Left: The pole-shaped electrosurgical probe is on the left and the tissue is on the right of the image. The probe is transmitting large amount of current into the tissue, which is seen to cause a high degree of resistive heat (diathermy) and results in a burn path through the tissue. These systems must be plugged into a wall outlet to provide sufficient electrical current for this process.
Right: High-magnification view of the process discussed above. We see the very end of the electrosurgical probe passing energy into the tissue on the right side of the image. In this schematic diagram, round black dots represent molecules and black lines represent the molecular bonds. In the area of the probe tip we see that the molecules and bonds are charred, twisted, and burnt, an effect that has been supported by academic histologic studies.

all present electrosurgical systems operate on a principle known as "diathermy." Standard electrosurgical systems do not operate by conditioning the emitted EM field to be highly absorbed by the matter in the intended path of the incision. Therefore, the EM field conducts through the body tissue as if it were passing through a poorly conductive wire. In this way, the EM field encounters a high degree of resistance, which creates resistive heat. This resistive heat causes the tissue to heat up and burn, thus creating a burn path in the tissue with charred margins (Fig. 2.4).

Let us now focus on how standard electrosurgery units operate. In simple terms, monopolar electrical cutting units have a hand piece and a collector plate that is placed somewhere on or near the body. In the case of bipolar forceps-style units, the hand piece has a jeweler-forceps configuration. The current is passed down one of the sides of the forceps then through the tissue and back up the other side of the forceps. These bipolar units, therefore, do not need a collector plate to collect the current, as monopolar units require. Most electrosurgical cutting units are a monopolar unit with a collecting plate design; thus, we will proceed to discuss this type of system. These monopolar systems emit conditioned EM fields from the blunt cutting tip with electronic modification such as rectification and filtration, which allow the surgeon to change the type of burn in tissue. Nonetheless, all modes produce heat, which causes a burn or cut with charred incision walls, a cauterizing (tissue-burning) hemostasis, or both. These types of systems produce an EM field that is transferred into tissue wherein it is poorly absorbed by the molecules and instead passes through the tissue as if the tissue were a wire that presents resistance. As the electrical energy passes through a resistive medium, it produces a great deal of heat. This is similar to the heat produced by friction—e.g., a drill bit grinding against a metal plate gets extremely hot. Keep in mind that the energy emitted by the electrosurgical unit is truly an EM field stream rather than a stream of electrons. However, this EM field will in turn react with electrons in the tissue in a manner that causes the electrons to pulse violently in the molecular lattice and thereby generate heat. The EM field travels at the speed of light, whereas the electrons in the tissue move in a random fashion at about 1/200 the speed of light. However, the movement of the electron through the tissue in a specific direction is minuscule, since the electrons bounce around the lattice of the molecular tissue like a ball bouncing randomly across the surface of a pinball machine. In a similar fashion, the filament of a light bulb is not an electron pipe; rather, the EM field that flows out of the wall outlet passes through the cable of the lamp then through the bulb filament. The EM field causes the electrons in the bulb filament to pulse forcefully such that they generate heat to a level at which light is given off. Therefore, the source of the electrons that cause an effect in both the tissue and the light bulb filament are from the electrons of the body tissue and the bulb filament itself. Electrons do not flow out of the wall electrical socket; rather, an EM field that flows at the speed of light flows out of the wall socket. This is similar to what occurs when surfers encounter a large wave, wherein the wave forces or pushes the surfer upward in a forceful pulsatile fashion for several seconds. The EM field does to the electrons in a bulb filament or in a tissue incision path precisely what an ocean wave does to the surfer. In both cases, the electron or the surfer is caused to accelerate, or pulse, for a short time. A high percentage of this energy transferred to the pulsed electron is converted into heat because of the resistive nature of the tissue. In summary, Figure 2.4 shows an EM field being discharged from the electrosurgical unit and into the body tissue, where it causes electrons in the tissue to pulse and thereby cause a resistive heat discharge sufficient to burn a path in the tissue. Therefore, the incision path is a burnt cavity with charred distorted walls.

The diagrams in Figure 2.5 show a laser beam on the left being focused on tissue, thereby creating a laser ablation path. Lasers are complicated, highly sensitive mechanisms that allow EM fields (i.e., light) to be focused on matter. EM fields are made up of small packets of energy called "photons" or "Planck EM quanta" (or PEQ). These photons are highly concentrated and focused by the laser such that they dramatically raise the energy level of the molecular lattice of the matter to a point at which it shatters into small pieces. Lasers suffer from high cost as well as control issues, making damage to adjacent structures an issue as well as reflected laser light causing foveal burns that result in blindness.

The diagrams in Figure 2.6 show the Fugo blade creating a plasma ablation path in tissue. The Fugo blade console looks grossly like a simple electrosurgical system, but actually functions similarly to a laser. The Fugo blade uses energy from batteries or a wall socket, then conditions, focuses, and concentrates the energy into an intense EM field that coats the blunt cutting filament. Unlike a standard electrosurgical system, the EM field of the Fugo blade is intensely absorbed by the matter in the intended path of incision. When the energy level of the matter exceeds the molecular bond energy, the molecules shatter. This is called the "photon bath theory" of ablation and occurs with the laser as well as the Fugo blade. When the intense EM field of the Fugo blade comes in contact with matter, it hyperexcites the molecules in the

Standard View

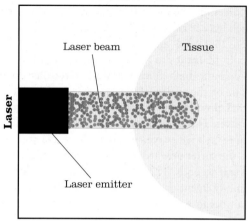

Laser Beam Reacting with Tissue

Ultrahigh-Magnification View

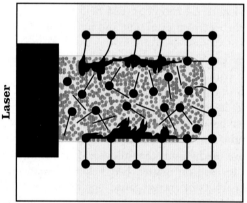

Laser Path Coated with Denatured Molecules and
Molecular Fragments in Center of Laser Beam

Figure 2.5. A diagram of laser cutting. **Left:** The laser is seen to project its coherent beam of EM field onto tissue. **Right:** A high-magnification view shows that the EM field of the laser makes an incision by causing a tissue disruption with involvement of molecules (round black dots) and molecular bonds (black lines).

Standard View

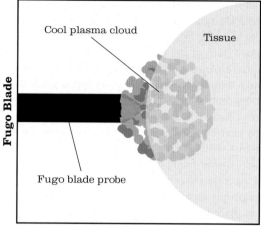

Plasma Field Reacting with Tissue

Ultrahigh-Magnification View

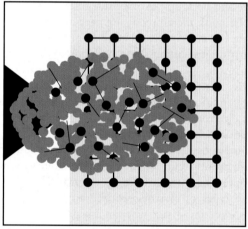

Cool Ablation Field with Molecular Fragments

Figure 2.6. A diagram of Fugo blade ablation cuts. **Left:** The round, blunt cutting probe of the Fugo blade on the left of the image is seen to create a cool plasma field where it contacts tissue. **Right:** A high-magnification view shows that the cool plasma field transmits energy, which is then absorbed by the molecular lattice of the tissue in the same way that EM fields are transmitted and absorbed by tissue as seen with the laser. Both laser and Fugo plasma ablation have the capability of creating pristine incision walls.

molecular lattice. The molecules then shatter into small fragments. These small fragments are absorbed into the intense focused EM field coating the blunt cutting filament of the Fugo blade. These small fragments are then used as the fuel for the plasma cloud of the Fugo blade.[5] By using the atomic particles in the path of the incision as the fuel for the plasma cloud, the Fugo blade creates "primary plasma," which has minimal impact on the tissue adjacent to the incision; therefore, this technique produces pristine incision walls.[6] On the other hand, older approaches that use fuels such as argon or propane generate "secondary plasma," which greatly damages tissue adjacent to the incision and therefore leaves charred, burnt incision walls.

The thickness of the plasma cloud in the Fugo blade can be changed from 50 μm to 75 μm to 100 μm by simply changing a switch on the Fugo blade console. The left-hand image in Figure 2.7 is an unfiltered image that demonstrates a thick, bright plume of light (not heat) surrounding the thin, inner plasma cloud. The center image in Figure 2.7 is a moderately filtered view of the activated plasma tip that filters away the large ball of light surrounding the inner core of plasma. Therefore, one can see the thin layer of

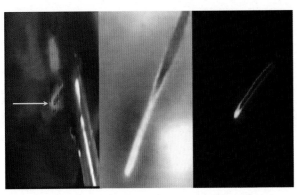

Figure 2.7. Plasma coating an activated Fugo blade ablation filament. **Left:** An unfiltered view of the plasma shows a thick ball of light (not heat) that surrounds the blunt ablation filament (*arrow*). **Center:** A moderately filtered image of the activated Fugo blade tip shows a thin coating of plasma over the blunt filament. This looks like a stick (cutting probe) that is dipped into honey (plasma). In real time, this coating is swirling in a controlled fashion at extremely high velocities. **Right:** A high-density filtered image of the activated Fugo blade tip shows only the thin coating of plasma, which has the highest energy density of all matter in this photo.

Scanning electron micrograph (SEM) images of the walls of incisions created by standard electrosurgery (diathermy) vs. Fugo Blade ablation

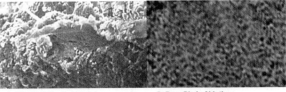

A: Standard Electrosurgery
Blistered, burnt, irregular and charred

B: Fugo Blade Ablation
Pristine clean incision walls

Figure 2.8. Scanning electron microscopy images of standard electrosurgery versus Fugo blade plasma ablation. **Left:** Standard diathermy is seen to cause incision walls to have a burnt, blistered, and cauterized surface. **Right:** Fugo blade ablation paths create pristine incision walls.

plasma that coats the blunt activated cutting tip. The right-hand image in Figure 2.7 is a dense filter image of the activated cutting tip wherein only the high-energy plasma field is visualized. Note the thin, bright layer of plasma that coats the blunt, activated cutting filament. In real time, plasma is highly dynamic, and therefore rapidly moves over the surface of the blunt cutting filament.

The Fugo blade system consists of an electronic console, a footswitch, and an ergonomic hand piece (Fig. 2.3). Unlike a diathermy unit, the hand piece of the Fugo blade contains internal electronics, and no collector plate must be placed on or near the patient. The Fugo blade is cleared by the FDA for anterior capsulotomy, transciliary filtration in glaucoma, and iridotomy for glaucoma, anterior chamber lenses or IOLs and ICLs. Each of the FDA clearances is a unique surgical procedure. The ophthalmic Fugo blade system performs all three procedures and is used worldwide. Many other surgical protocols are underway in and outside ophthalmology. The hand piece is sterilized in the same tray as the phaco hand piece. The unit is simple to maintain and use.

Academic evaluation of the Fugo blade includes numerous clinical trials, as well as studies of histology and biomechanics. Some of the finest academic histologic studies include scanning electron micrographs of the wall of the capsulotomy created with Fugo blade plasma ablation. Also, high-resolution microscopy of

Fugo blade plasma blade ablation paths in rabbit corneas were performed at Louisiana State University.[6] Dr. David Apple's group performed microscopy on Fugo blade capsulotomy rims and demonstrated that the Fugo blade produces the highly desirable "postage stamp margin" for capsulotomies.[7] The basic findings from all these studies demonstrate that Fugo blade plasma ablation produces pristine incision walls, whereas diathermy produces charred, burnt, and irregular incision walls (Fig. 2.8). This is immensely important on a clinical level, since a clean incision wall eliminates the need for the breakdown and removal of charred debris, which delays healing, causes redness and swelling, and increases pain in soft-tissue incisions.

Biomechanical studies of the strength of the capsulotomy rim were performed at the University of South Carolina. This study demonstrates that the capsulotomy rim created with the Fugo blade was stronger than all other techniques, including diathermy, except for capsulorrhexis.[7] A graph of different capsulotomy techniques has been generated based on the University of South Carolina data and is shown in Figure 2.9.[8–10] Capsulorrhexis is the strongest capsulotomy rim because the Fugo blade ablates pristine capsulotomy walls wherever the surgeon traces or moves the ablation filament, and thereby does not stay within natural tissue planes of the anterior capsule. On the other hand, capsulorrhexis is a tearing of the anterior capsule, which stays within natural tissue planes. Once a capsulorrhexis escapes from the natural tissue planes of the anterior capsule, it has a high risk of tearing out into the periphery. A capsulorrhexis tear will continue to tear until it is completed because the head of the capsulorrhexis is an acute angle. Meanwhile, the Fugo blade ablation path creates round ends; therefore, they will not continue to tear spontaneously under normal stress. Nonetheless, a lysis of tissue in natural tissue planes usually provides capsulotomy rims that are

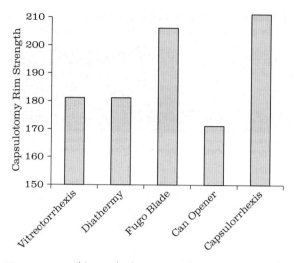

Figure 2.9. This graph shows capsulotomy rim strength based on various surgical techniques. This graph was generated from data that was compiled at the University of South Carolina, as discussed in the text. Note that the Fugo blade capsulotomy rim is significantly stronger than diathermy and is almost comparable to capsulorrhexis.

stronger than lysis of tissue that are not within natural tissue planes. However, the Fugo blade allows the surgeon to make the capsulotomy as large as desired in a safe, controlled fashion. By increasing the capsulotomy from 5 mm to 7 mm, we decrease the force on the capsulotomy rim by 33%, which gives a Fugo blade capsulotomy a big advantage over capsulorrhexis.

Several clinical features of Fugo blade plasma ablation provide distinct advantages over prior methods of tissue incision.[11] These features include:

Resistance-free incision. Plasma ablation is a method of "erasing" tissue, thereby acting like a miniature eximer laser because it converts tissue into a mist of water vapor and aromatic molecular fragments. Plasma ablation eliminates jerky, uncontrolled incising motions, which present a danger during surgery.

Pristine incision walls without cauterization. A pristine incision wall eliminates the tissues' need to mount a process to break down necrotic debris then remove the debris from the incision cavity. This is why plasma ablation provides quicker healing, less redness and swelling, less risk of infection, and less pain.

A noncauterizing hemostasis. Histologic studies have shown that the plasma ablation walls of the Fugo blade are pristine without cautery, yet clinical studies have shown that the Fugo blade produces hemostasis—a noncauterizing hemostasis. All other electrosurgical systems produce cauterizing hemostasis. Prior studies have demonstrated that

exposure of blood to plasma stimulates hemostasis. Plasma exposure stimulates platelet plug formation, which secretes serotonin and epinephrine to constrict the vessel wall as well as factors that stimulate the coagulation cascade. Thus, plasma stimulates noncauterizing hemostasis.

Antimicrobial activity. Infectious particles including viruses and prions are killed by exposure to plasma. Therefore, Fugo blade plasma ablation serves to disinfect while creating an incision path. This provides a significant advantage in reducing postoperative infection.

In conclusion, the Fugo plasma blade is the first paradigm shift in surgical incision since the introduction of the laser in the mid-1900s. This chapter has explained the biophysics of the Fugo blade as compared with other methods of incision. We have attempted to explain the novel capabilities of plasma ablation surgery, which has the potential to allow surgical procedures that were not possible with older technologies.

References

1. Fugo RJ, DelCampo DM. The Fugo blade™: the next step after capsulorrhexis. *Ann Ophthalmol.* 2001; 33:12–20.
2. Sabbagh LB. The leading edge: harnessing electrons for a faster, smarter incision. *Eyeworld.* 1998;3:88.
3. Video journal of cataract and refractive surgery. *New Developments New Devices Fugo Blade.* 2002;18(1).
4. Singh SK. Fugo blade capsulotomy: a new high tech cutting technology. *Trop Ophthalmol.* 2001;1:14–16.
5. Ronge L. How to use the Fugo blade. *EyeNet.* 2003; 7:23–24.
6. Peponis V, Rosenberg P, Reddy SV, et al. Study finds Fugo blade can be of use in corneal surgery. *Rev Ophthalmol.* 2006;8:94.
7. Izak AM, Werner L, Pandey SK, et al. Analysis of the capsule edge after Fugo plasma blade capsulotomy, continuous curvilinear capsulorrhexis, and can-opener capsulotomy. *J Cataract Refract Surg.* 2004;30:2606–2611.
8. Wilson ME, Trivedi RH. Technological advances make pediatric cataract surgery safer and faster. *Tech Ophthalmol.* 2003;1:53–61.
9. Wilson ME. Anterior lens capsule management in pediatric cataract surgery. *Trans Am Ophthalmol Soc.* 2004;102:391–422.
10. Trivedi RH, Wilson ME Jr, Bartholomew LR. Extensibility and scanning electron microscopy evaluation of 5 pediatric anterior capsulotomy techniques in a porcine model. *J Cataract Refract Surg.* 2006;32:1206–1213.
11. Singh D, Singh RSJ. Applications of the Fugo blade. In: Wilson ME Jr, Trivedi RH, Pandey SK, eds. *Pediatric cataract surgery; techniques, complications, and management.* Philadelphia, Pa: Lippincott, Williams & Wilkins, 2005:97–100.

Section II
Clinical Applications of the Fugo Blade

Part A
The Eyelid–Lacrimal System

Conjunctival Route Levator Plication for Ptosis

DALJIT SINGH

P tosis has many causes. One convenient classification is infantile ptosis and adult ptosis. Ptosis is an indication for conjunctival-route levator plication, whether the ptosis is mild, moderate, or severe. The Fugo blade's ability to incise and blunt-dissect bloodlessly encouraged me to look for the levator muscle through fornix incisions and to advance the blade to the anterior surface of the tarsal plate. This new technique is called "sutureless conjunctival-route plication of the levator" or simply "Singh levator plication." (The conjunctival entry incisions are sutureless; however, levator plication requires buried sutures.)

Plication can be performed in both infantile and adult ptosis. Most cases of ptosis are uniocular, but in bilateral ptosis, I prefer to do one eye at a time. Plication may or may not work for paralytic ptosis. It is useful for cases of Marcus Gunn ptosis, because the correction of ptosis reduces the range of jaw-wink lid excursion.

TECHNIQUE

Anesthesia

During surgery, double eversion must be performed on the eyelid must undergo double eversion to create considerable pull on the lid. Pull on the muscle is produced as the levator is located, grasped, and brought forward. Because of this, I prefer to give general anesthesia, even for adults.

Surgical Technique

1. Perform double eversion of the lid using a Desmarre lid retractor (Fig. 3.1).

2. Pass thick nylon stay sutures through at the upper edge of the tarsal plate, one in the center

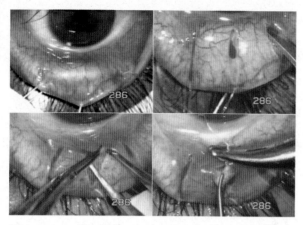

Figure 3.1. The lid has undergone double eversion with a Desmarre lid retractor. Thick nylon stay sutures are passed close to the upper edge of the tarsal plate. The conjunctiva is ballooned with lignocaine, and three vertical conjunctival incisions are made using the Fugo blade. The Müller muscle is pulled anteriorly so that the levator can be grasped. An anchoring suture is passed through the levator muscle.

and one on each side at a distance of about 6 mm. The weight of the artery forceps holding the sutures keeps the lid everted.

3. Use lignocaine 2% to balloon the conjunctiva over the double-everted tarsus.

4. Make three conjunctival vertical incisions about 10 mm long in line with the stay sutures using a 100-μm Fugo blade tip. When this tip crosses a large subconjunctival vessel, bleeding occurs. To prevent this ablate/close all visible blood vessels in the proposed line of incision using a 300-μm tip at low energy. Alternatively, you may start and complete the incision using the 300-μm tip only. This leaves a minor gap in the conjunctiva, which does not affect the surgical result.

5. The fornix ends of the conjunctival incisions are undermined toward the orbit.

6. The structure directly beneath the incised conjunctiva is Müller muscle, which originates beneath the levator muscle is better and deep to this is the levator muscle. If you pull this muscle anteriorly, the levator muscle can be caught easily in its aponeurosis. Whereas the Müller muscle is red, the levator muscle appears pearly white. The amount of levator muscle you should pull anteriorly depends on the severity of ptosis: The greater the ptosis, the more anteriorly you should pull the levator muscle.

7. Pass an 80-μm vanadium steel suture through the levator muscle caught at the end of each conjunctival incision and secure the sutures with miniclamps.

8. Expose the anterior surface of the tarsal plate using a 300-μm blunt Fugo blade probe. Expose the surface at the three proximal ends of the conjunctival incisions. Expose the tarsal plate as ablation of the Müller muscle and the underlying stretched aponeurosis of the levator muscle. Start ablation close to the nylon stay sutures, which provide a clue to the depth at which the Fugo blade is working. The most important point is not to ablate the tarsal plate, but only to expose it. Tarsal plate exposure with the Fugo blade is usually bloodless, but if a large vessel is in the way, it will bleed. You can touch the same Fugo blade tip to the bleeding spot to stop the bleeding. Exposing the tarsal plate using the Fugo blade does not burn the tissues, preventing postoperative reaction and edema (Fig. 3.2).

9. Next, pass the steel sutures that are holding the levator muscle through the exposed/prepared anterior surface of the tarsal plate. Insert the needle through a partial thickness of the tarsal plate, about 3 to 3.5 mm from the upper edge of the plate, and exit about 1.5 mm from the edge.

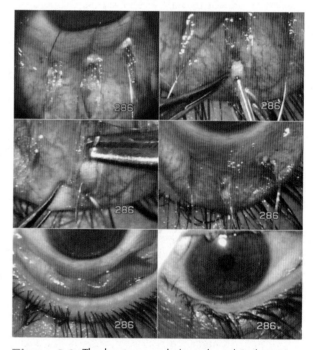

Figure 3.2. The levator muscle is anchored at three points with sutures. The anterior surface of the tarsal is carefully exposed at three places with a 300-μm Fugo blade tip. The levator anchoring sutures are passed through the half thickness of the tarsal plate, at about 3.5 mm from the upper edge of the tarsal plate, then the sutures are tied, and the lid is returned to the normal position. No conjunctival sutures are required.

10. Attach the levator muscle to the tarsal plate with a reef knot in the steel sutures. Do not use excessive force to pull the sutures, or they may cut through the tissue.

11. Remove the stay sutures and return the lid to its normal position. When the lid is in its normal position, the sutures are situated on the anterior surface of the tarsal plate, i.e., they do not face the cornea or the bulbar conjunctiva.

12. Temporarily tie the lids together with a thick nylon suture—24 hours for adults and 48 hours for children.

Note that the Fugo blade is needed for the critical steps of incising the conjunctiva and exposing the anterior surface of the tarsal plate. Do not attempt to make a lid fold; the lid fold naturally occurs.

Postoperative Management

Direct the patient to apply steroid-antibiotic eye ointment three times a day for 15 days and instill artificial tear drops seven to eight times a day for 15 days. Make sure that the patient is able to close the lid. Advise the patient that a pad and bandage should be used overnight or while sleeping for the first few days.

Little or no inflammatory reaction occurs after this surgery, partly because the Fugo blade ablates the tissue without charring it and partly because of the simplicity and atraumatic nature of the surgical technique.

It is important to watch the lid margin for any turning in. This can happen if the levator muscle is attached too far anteriorly from the superior edge of the tarsal plate. Turning in can also occur in very severe ptosis, for which an excess of levator muscle must be pulled out. In this case, the tarsal plate moves up, while the other tissues of the lid tend to hang over the lid margin. Temporary sutures that lift the skin prevent the cilia from striking the cornea. A bandage lens may be worn for a few days if needed.

Summary

My colleagues and I have performed more than 180 of these levator plication operations during the past 5 years. We have had a satisfactory outcome in more than 90% of the cases. When the correction does not meet expectations, we perform additional surgery using plication of the orbicularis oculi muscle. A waiting period of about 3 to 4 months is needed before a second surgery can be done. Examples of some of our results are shown in Figures 3.3, 3.4, and 3.5.

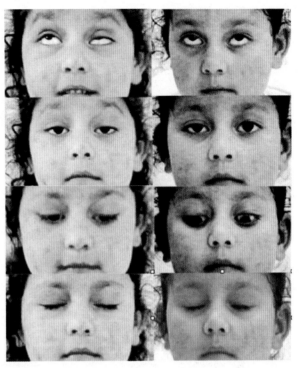

Figure 3.3. A pediatric patient with ptosis in both eyes, and more severe in the left eye. The photos show the patient's preoperative (**Left**) and 1 month postoperative (**Right**) appearance while looking up, looking straight, looking down, and closing her eyes. Lid lag, but no lagophthalmos, is present while looking down.

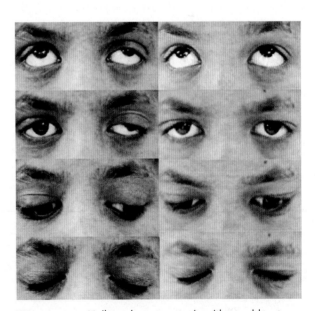

Figure 3.4. Unilateral severe ptosis with good levator function in a 13-year-old patient. The postoperative appearances (**Right**) are 1 year after the operation. Lid lag, but no lagophthalmos, is present in the operated eye.

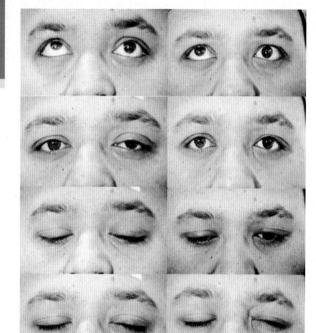

Figure 3.5. Residual ptosis after a Fasanella–Servat operation on the left eye. Poor elevation of the left eye was a pre-existing condition. The preoperative and 1 week postoperative results, after levator plication, are shown. The operated eye can be closed easily.

In 1981, Beard stated "All told . . . well over a hundred operations and variations of operations for ptosis have been reported. This is good evidence that the 'ideal' operation has not as yet been devised and probably never shall be. Our present concepts may seem archaic in the not too distant future."[1] About Müller muscle, Beard writes in his preface, "Here is a structure of obvious importance that has been largely disregarded by many of us. This muscle has been ruthlessly excised in many levator resections. It could be that ptosis surgery in the future will be largely aimed at the preservation of this structure. . . ."

Our goal has been to develop a ptosis surgery technique that:

- involves minimal handling of tissues,
- preserves the Müller muscle,
- may be redone to reduce or enhance the correction,
- does not compromise the ocular tissues for additional surgery by any other currently used surgical technique,
- is applicable to all grades of ptosis, and
- is easy to learn.

Our experience shows that all the points mentioned above are more or less achieved by our technique. Hence, we believe that this new concept of "sutureless plication of levator muscle" is a step toward the realization of an ideal ptosis procedure. The Fugo blade is a major ally in performing the most crucial steps of the procedure in a bloodless manner.

Suggested Reading

Agatson SA. Resection of levator palpebrae muscle by the conjunctival route for ptosis. *Arch Ophthalmol.* 1942;27:994.

Beard C. *Ptosis.* St. Louis, Mo: Mosby, 1981.

Berke RN. A simplified Blaskovics operation for blepharoptosis. *Arch Ophthalmol.* 1954;48:460.

Blaskovics L. A new operation for ptosis with shortening of the levator and tarsus. *Arch Ophthalmol.* 1923;52:563.

Cohen AJ. Ptosis, adult. Accessed January 3, 2010, at http://www.emedicine.com/oph/topic201.htm.

Iliff CE. A simplified ptosis operation. *Am J Ophthalmol.* 1954;37:529.

Roy FH. Ptosis: complete classification. *Ann Ophthalmol.* 2005;37:5–32.

Singh D, Fugo RJ. Orbicularis plication for ptosis, a third alternative. *Ann Ophthalmol.* 2006;38:185–193.

Singh D, Kaur A, Singh K, et al. Sutureless levator plication by conjunctival route: a new technique. *Ann Ophthalmol.* 2006;38:285–292.

Suh DW. Ptosis, congenital. Accessed January 3, 2010, at http://www.emedicine.com/oph/topic345.htm.

Trichiasis DALJIT SINGH and KIRANJIT SINGH

The anterior portion of the eyelid contains the lashes embedded in hair follicles. In some instances, a lash can point toward the eye. This condition is called "trichiasis." Trichiasis without entropion must be treated by destroying the roots of the individual cilia.

According to Elders[1] the dimensions of the follicles are (mean ±SD): upper lid follicle depth, 1.8±0.3 mm; bulb width, 188±44 μm; shaft width, 205±28 μm; lower lid follicle depth, 0.9±0.2 mm; bulb width 132±19 μm; and shaft width, 158±26 μm. Significant differences exist in the anatomy of the follicles between the two lids. For an electrolysis needle to completely contact 95% of all follicles, it must be inserted 2.4 mm into the upper lid and 1.4 mm into the lower lid.

The causes of lash misdirection are numerous, and some are listed in Table 4.1. The most common among

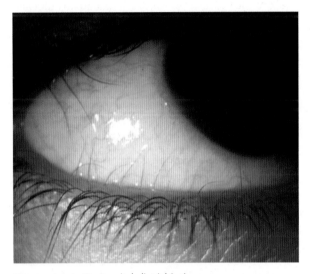

Figure 4.1. Congenital districhiasis.

these are trachoma, Steven–Johnson syndrome, and trauma. When trichiasis is accompanied by entropion, both the lid and the lashes must be treated. In congenital districhiasis (Fig. 4.1), an extra row of small eyelashes abnormally grow on the inner surface or very edge of the eyelids. Both upper and lower lids may be involved. This leads to epiphora and hazy vision. Each individual cilium must be dealt with.

Regardless of the cause, when errant eyelashes touch the cornea, treatment is indicated.

TECHNIQUE

Many procedures have been described for the treatment of trichiasis: simple epilation, electrolysis, cryosurgery, argon-laser ablation, and radiofrequency ablation. But

Table 4.1. Common Causes of Trichiasis

Cause	Example
Infectious	Trachoma Herpes zoster
Autoimmune	Ocular cicatricial pemphigoid
Inflammatory	Stevens–Johnson syndrome Vernal keratoconjunctivitis
Trauma, postsurgical	Lower lid transconjunctival approach for floor fracture repair or blepharoplasty After enucleation After ectropion repair
Trauma, chemical	Alkali burns to the eye
Thermal burns to face/lids	
Congenital districhiasis	

epilation is a temporary measure, electrolysis is tedious, and cryosurgery has potential problems as damaging additional hair follicles. Radiofrequency ablation is effective; the core tissue is removed by the cut–coagulate method. A lot of energy is transferred to the tissue in the process, however, which produces tissue reaction and some scarring. The Fugo blade is swift and highly effective for cilia removal. It does so swiftly and effectively. The technique could be termed the "fugolysis" of cilia.

The figures 4.2, 4.3, 4.4, and 4.5 record the treatment of a patient with Steven–Johnson syndrome in who a new row of cilia had developed as a result of metaplasia of the meibomian glands.

Anesthesia

Prepare the patient by injecting adequate lidocaine along the lid margin.

Surgical Technique

Several Fugo blade tips are available. I use either a 3.5-mm naked (without insulating tubing) 100-μm Fugo blade tip or a long, tapered 300-μm tip.

1. Use medium power and energy settings for destroying the cilia roots.

2. Align the tip with the cilium. Slip the ablating tip alongside the shaft of the cilium (Fig. 4.2). (If the misdirected cilia are short, stiff, and tight in the tissue and do not allow a 100-μm tip to enter alongside the shaft, use a sharp, pointed 300-μm tip; it performs just as well as the 100-μm tip.)

3. When the tip reaches the desired depth, activate it momentarily (Fig. 4.3). For the tip to be

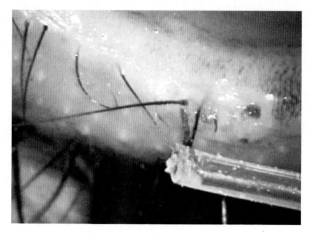

Figure 4.3. The tip is activated when it reaches the depth of the follicle.

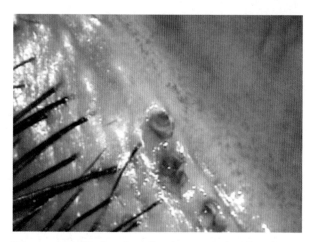

Figure 4.4. No burning effect is seen at the site where ablation has been carried out.

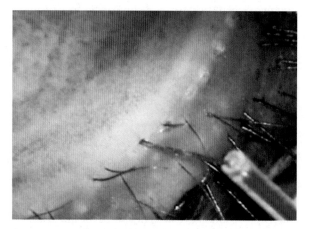

Figure 4.2. The naked 100-μm fiber of the Fugo blade tip is slipped alongside the cilium.

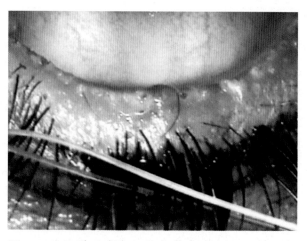

Figure 4.5. The whole row of cilia have been removed.

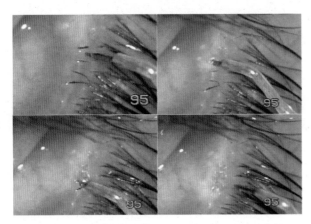

Figure 4.6. A 300-μm tapered tip has been used to ablate the cilia roots in this case.

effective, it should reach the root of the cilia for ablation.

4. As you withdraw the inactivated tip, the cilium comes along with it.

The procedure is extremely quick. You can confidently remove a whole row of cilia in congenital districhiasis in a couple of minutes. You can remove the core tissue by ablation using minimal energy transfer through resonance. No burning or coagulation of the tissues is involved (Figs. 4.4–4.6).

Postoperative Management

This procedure does not cause postoperative pain or scarring. If a follicle fails to be destroyed, the procedure can be repeated.

Reference

1. Elders MJ. Anatomy and physiology of eyelash follicles: relevance to lash ablation. *Ophthalmol Plast Reconstr Surg.* 1997;13:21–25.

5 Sebaceous Cyst SEEMA K SINGH

A sebaceous cyst is caused by obstruction of the gland of Zeiss, the meibomian gland, or the sebaceous glands associated with the hair follicles of the eyelid. Sebaceous cysts are solid white or yellowish and present like a tumor beneath the normal skin. The consistency is soft to rubbery.

The standard surgical procedure is to make an incision larger than the diameter of the cyst. Blunt dissection is then done to separate the cyst from the surrounding tissues, and the cyst is removed completely. Bleeding is controlled with cautery, excess skin is excised, and the skin is closed with nylon or silk sutures or absorbable sutures.

CASE STUDY

We treated a 70-year-old patient who had a large (9 mm) sebaceous cyst along the lid margin close to the punctum. A normal surgical procedure could have jeopardized the function of the punctum. Therefore, we took the steps outlined below to remove the cyst.

TECHNIQUE

Anesthesia

Infiltrate lidocaine around the cyst.

Surgical Technique

1. Incise the cyst wall very carefully with a 100-μm Fugo blade tip set at the lowest energy levels. The incision should be full length. The contents of the cyst will be visible under the incision (Fig. 5.1).

2. Use a plane forceps to hold the cyst at the deepest point, then move the forceps upward, to squeeze out and drain the contents of the cyst. A part of the cyst wall also appears; it should also be pulled out.

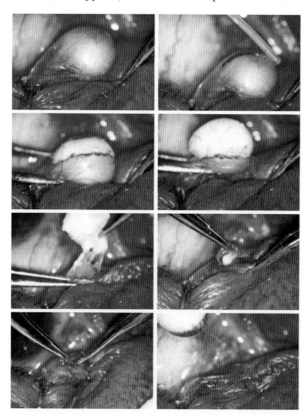

Figure 5.1. A cyst close to the punctum is incised with the Fugo blade. The contents are squeezed out with plain forceps. The wall of the cyst is pulled out. Excess skin is excised. No suture is applied.

3. Pull out the visible cyst wall inside the cyst cavity using a fine forceps.

4. Excise the loose excess skin. Because the skin edges are naturally approximated, do not apply sutures. If the incision is particularly long, however, a couple of sutures may be needed.

Summary

Even the most minor-looking ailment needs the best attention, even if it does not threaten the patient's vision. The cosmetic sensitivity of lesions on the face and especially near the eye demands the least traumatic approach. The Fugo blade is of help in these situations because it can make incisions and remove tissues without burning and charring the adjacent tissue.

Suggested Reading

Kellan R, Fugo RJ. Device increases safety, efficiency of cataract surgery. *Ophthalmol Times.* 2000;25(22):7–9.
Roy FH. Course of Fugo blade is enlightening, surgeon says. *Ocular Surg News.* 2001;19:35–38.

6

Dysfunction of the Meibomian Glands DALJIT SINGH

The term *anterior blepharitis* refers to inflammation of the eyelashes and follicles. *Posterior blepharitis* refers to meibomian gland dysfunction. Blepharitis often is associated with systemic diseases such as rosacea, as well as ocular diseases such as the dry eye syndrome, conjunctivitis, and keratitis. Many patients have a history of a drug reaction or fever associated with their blepharitis.

Patients with posterior blepharitis have ocular symptoms of burning, watering, foreign-body sensation, photophobia, and decreased vision.

On examination, you may find crusting of the lashes and meibomian orifices and plugging and "pouting" of the meibomian orifices. Corneal findings can include punctuate epithelial erosions and corneal ulcers or pannus.

Posterior blepharitis is related to dysfunction of the meibomian glands; the meibomian secretions become waxlike and block the gland orifices. Visual inspection reveals the typical plugging and "pouting" of the meibomian orifices, leading to diagnosis. Test for tear insufficiency aids in diagnosis, leading to improved dry eye treatment.

Early in these conditions, we recommend the following treatment:

1. Hot packs to the lids. The goal is to get the secretions in the meibomian glands to melt, liquefy, and drain out to the lid margin.

2. A balanced diet rich in fruits and vitamins.

3. A teaspoonful of flaxseed oil every day. We have found that flaxseed oil ameliorates many symptoms. A drop in the eye also helps.

If the condition is advanced and medical treatment is not working, surgery is recommended. Surgery in these cases consists of opening each individual meibomian duct. This procedure can be accomplished with the Fugo blade, which opens the ducts without charring or burning tissue. Before the advent of the Fugo blade, there was no device that could perform this function.

Both lids of one eye are treated at the first sitting, so that the patient can compare the relief obtained from the operation with the condition of the untreated eye. The worst eye is treated first.

TECHNIQUE

Anesthesia

Use topical anesthetic and lidocaine along the lid margin.

Surgical Technique

1. Use either the standard capsulotomy Fugo plasma blade tip or a special sharp pointed long tip (300 μm) (Fig. 6.1). The idea is to clear the meibomian ducts and not damage the glands. Apply the lowest energy settings for ablation.

2. Control the position of the lid margin with the thumb, such that the openings of the meibomian ducts are available for vertical penetration.

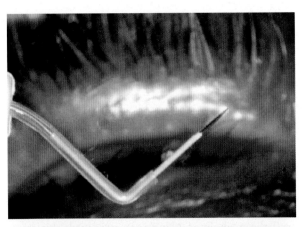

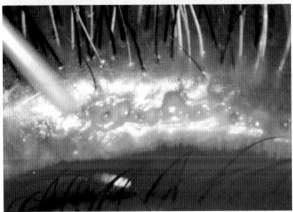

Figure 6.1. A long, sharp, pointed Fugo blade tip outside and inside the meibomian gland.

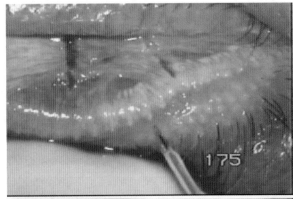

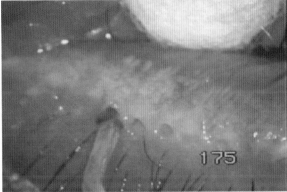

Figure 6.2. Heavily plugged meibomian gland openings before and during treatment.

3. Align the tip vertically, activate it, and insert it into the meibomian duct. When a duct is treated, a fatty substance flows out. When the tip is withdrawn a small gaping hole is left where earlier the fatty plug was (Figs. 6.2 and 6.3). We often see secretions coming out of the adjoining meibomian openings, which may indicate the presence of communicating channels between adjacent glands.

4. Treat each meibomian gland in 1 to 2 seconds, so that all the glands are treated within a short time.

Postoperative Management

Advise patients that during the postoperative period they should continue with hot packs at least twice a day, maintain a nourishing diet, and take a spoonful of flaxseed oil daily.

Prescribe artificial tears as needed for burning or tearing and oil-based lubricant/antibiotics once or twice a day.

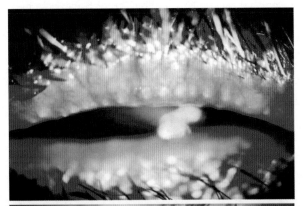

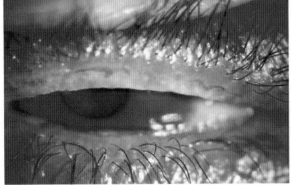

Figure 6.3. Secretion-plugged meibomian glands before and 4 hours after Fugo blade treatment.

6

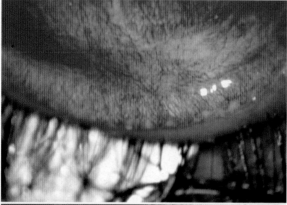

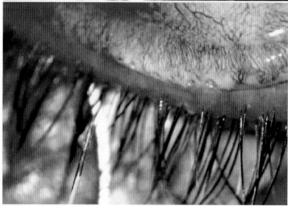

Figure 6.4. Finely plugged meibomian gland openings before and after treatment with the Fugo blade. Note the absence of burning or charring.

Patients commonly feel relief within 3 to 4 hours of meibomian gland treatment. No burning or charring of tissue occurs (Fig. 6.4). In most patients, the need for local artificial tears is greatly reduced and or even eliminated. Our patients are advised to return every 2 months, as some of them require retreatment.

Summary

During the past 5 years we have treated more than 20 patients with this method. Every patient benefitted to some extent from the treatment. The operation reduced their dependence on artificial tears. We advise patients to avoid being in the sun, especially in the summer, and to reduce evaporation of tears by closing their eyes for a few minutes every now and then.

If the meibomian glands are atrophied, this treatment does not help to improve secretion of the glands. However, the irritation and gritty feeling from the plugs at the lid margins is eliminated.

Patients with Stevens–Johnson syndrome may exhibit symptoms of meibomian gland dysfunction, not only plugged meibomian glands but also metaplasia, so that cilia grow from the meibomian ducts. These conditions can be treated with the Fugo blade.

Many people live with the terrible reality of dry eyes and are totally dependent on the frequent use of artificial tears. Some of these patients' conditions are suitable for treatment of meibomian glands using the Fugo blade. For these patients, it is wise to proceed cautiously by treating only a few glands at a time and observing the response.

Suggested Reading

Cohen EJ. Cornea and external disease in the new millennium. *Arch Ophthalmol.* 2000;118:979–981.

Lowery RS. Adult blepharitis. Accessed January 3, 2010, at www.emedicine.com/oph/topic81.htm.

Tarsorrhaphy SEEMA K. SINGH

F acial palsy, which usually affects only one side of the face, is a primary indication for tarsorrhaphy. In facial palsy, the blink reflex is affected and the front surface of the eye may dry out. When this occurs, tarsorrhaphy is indicated to partially close the eye to protect the cornea.

Tarsorrhaphy is not a simple procedure. Failed surgeries are common because the tarsal plates of the two lids often do not join as expected.

We have devised a procedure that uses stainless steel sutures to bring the tissues together. Raw areas on the lid margins are created using the Fugo blade. The Fugo blade offers a distinct advantage over manual incisions because it produces little or no bleeding.

TECHNIQUE

Anesthesia

Infiltrate the upper and lower lids with 2% lidocaine.

Surgical Technique

1. Bring together the upper and lower lids where they are to be joined. Pass a stout nylon suture through both lids (Fig. 7.1). This secures and steadies the lids for the surgical steps to follow.

2. Use a 100-μm Fugo blade tip, set at the lowest energy setting, to make two incisions on the inter-

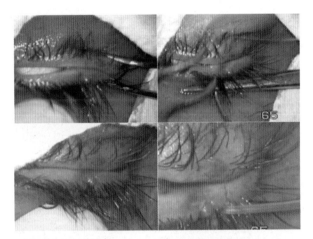

Figure 7.1. The upper and lower lids are held together with a stout forceps as a thick nylon suture is passed across both lids and secured. **Bottom right:** Two vertical incisions are made on both lids with the Fugo blade.

marginal strip of each lid. Make the incisions about 5 mm apart and less than 1 mm deep.

3. Incise the intermarginal strip between the two incisions and gently lift as a flap, starting from the side of the posterior lid margin and proceeding toward the ciliary edge. The flap may be about ¾ mm thick. Take care not to point the Fugo blade anteriorly, which would immediately cut the flap. Treat both lids the same way. The result is a flap each on the two lids and a raw strip of tarsal plate underneath, perfectly aligned (Fig. 7.2).

4. Join together the two raw areas of the lid margins as follows. Pass an 80-μm vanadium steel suture from the raw side outward to a short distance from the cilia. Then reverse the suture and pass

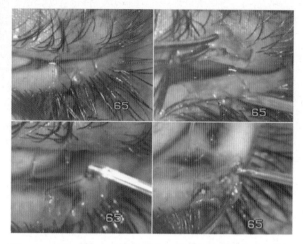

Figure 7.2. After making all four incisions, the lower lid flap has been made. A similar flap is then made in the upper lid.

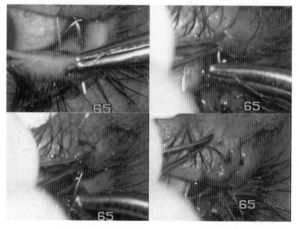

Figure 7.3. The 80-μm stainless steel suture is passed upward through the raw area of the upper lid and is then passed through the skin. The needle is passed through the raw area of the lower lid, then returned from the skin side. The two ends of the suture are tied, bringing the raw areas together.

it from the skin to the raw area side. Repeat these steps in the opposite lid and pass the suture back through the raw areas (Fig. 7.3).

5. Now, with one loop of vanadium steel sutures in each lid, use the two ends of the suture to bring the raw areas together. Tie the suture as a reef knot, taking care not to let the marginal flaps get in the way, and cut the suture close to the knot. The knot at this point is covered by the free marginal flaps. The suture becomes buried in the skin and causes no inflammation (Fig. 7.4).

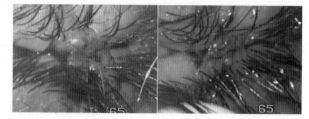

Figure 7.4. Left: The 80-μm vanadium steel suture has been tied off. The suture is then cut under the flaps. **Right:** The 40-μm vanadium steel sutures have been applied, thus completing the operation.

6. Suture the flaps from the two lids with 40-μm vanadium steel sutures. Two or three sutures are sufficient.

7. Remove the temporary nylon suture holding the lids together.

For temporary tarsorrhaphy, you can join the lids with 80-μm vanadium steel sutures without creating raw areas on the lid margins.

Postoperative Management

1. Remove the dressing after 3 hours.
2. Prescribe local antibiotic drops, to be instilled five to six times a day for 15 days.

Summary

Failures with this operation are rare and are usually related to making insufficient flaps, poor suturing, or the use of sutures other than steel. Within days, the main supporting 80-μm steel suture becomes completely buried, as it cuts through the skin under the loops. It need never be removed. Similarly, the 40-μm sutures to the flaps never need to be removed.

Suggested Reading

Beyer-Machule CK. Malposition of lids. In: Heilman, K, Palon, D, eds. *Atlas of ophthalmic surgery*. New York, NY: Thieme, 1985:1.36–1.37.

Iliff NT. Surgery of the eyelids and lacrimal drainage apparatus. In: Rice TA, Michels RG, Stark WJ, eds. *Ophthalmic surgery*. St. Louis, Mo: Mosby, 1984:40–41.

Roy FH. *Master techniques in ophthalmic surgery*. Baltimore, Md: Williams & Wilkins, 1985:740–741.

Congenital or Acquired Punctal Atresia and Canaliculus Closure

DALJIT SINGH

The medial ends of both the superior and the inferior lids contain a punctum. The puncta are situated on a slightly elevated platform, called the "lacrimal papillae," and face posteriorly, so it is necessary to evert the medial lids to inspect them. The lower punctum is more effective for draining tears.

Punctual stenosis may be congenital or acquired. Congenital punctal closure may be caused by a membrane on the punctum, or it may be a part of more extensive atresia. The use of local antiviral or antiglaucoma medication or local cicatrizing diseases of the conjunctiva may result in obstructions. An infrequent cause of functional closure of the punctum is enlargement of the caruncle that lies between the punctum and the lacus lacrimalis.

A dilator may be used to open a functionally closed punctum with soft elastic walls, but it may close shortly afterward because of the peculiar elasticity of the tissues. Patients with this condition are often frustrated because although syringing is always successful, they continue to suffer from epiphora.

Forcible dilation of the punctum usually fails. Unless some tissue in the mouth and the adjoining wall of the punctum is removed, the condition does not resolve. The treatments available for punctual closure are simple dilation, redilation, and posterior wall punctectomy, in which the vertical limb of the canaliculus is amputated. Because the failure rate is high, many ophthalmologists are reluctant to manage cases of punctal closure.

Treatment of Punctal Atresia

Acquired Punctal Atresia

In cases of functional blockage with no lid abnormality, the management is as outlined below.

TECHNIQUE

Anesthesia

Infiltrate lidocaine 2% near the lid margin and use surface anesthesia.

Surgical Technique

1. Insert the dilator into the punctum to confirm its position (Fig. 8.1). When you remove the dilator, the opening closes again, as expected. Syringe the area to confirm that the rest of the passage is clear.

2. Insert a medium-sized lacrimal probe into the punctum to reach the ampulla and hold it there.

3. Activate a 300-μm Fugo blade tip at the highest energy level and repeatedly touch it to the lacrimal probe at some distance away from the flesh. The tip

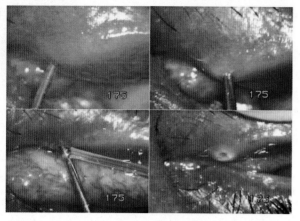

Figure 8.1. The punctum is hardly visible, but it easily accommodates a medium-size probe. The dilator is passed into the punctum. The probe is inserted into the ampulla. The activated Fugo blade tip touches the probe close to its entry point. A nice punctum is produced at the end of the procedure.

of the lacrimal probe actually performs the function of the Fugo blade tip every time it is touched, thereby trimming the tissue around the probe.

4. When you remove the lacrimal probe, a beautiful round punctum remains.

If the condition recurs, it is easy to repeat the treatment.

Postoperative Management

Infiltrate lidocaine 2% near the lid margin and use surface anesthesia.

Congenital Punctal Atresia

In congenital punctal atresia, the punctum may not be visible, or it may be seen vaguely or may appear as a shallow avascular spot or depression. Its presumed location is medial to the meibomian gland orifices. The inferior punctum is temporally displaced relative to the superior punctum, rather than lying directly across from it. The management of congenital atresia is somewhat different from that for acquired punctal atresia.

TECHNIQUE

Anesthesia

Infiltrate lidocaine 2% near the lid margin and use surface anesthesia.

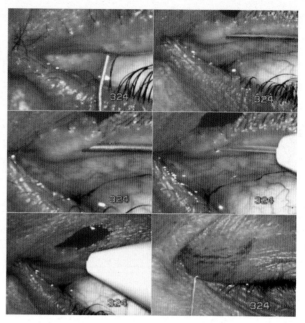

Figure 8.2. The canaliculus is visible as a grey line medial to the punctum. A thin probe encounters the obstruction. A thicker probe is inserted to dilate the canaliculus, through which a 300-μm soft Fugo blade tip is gently pushed up to the obstruction. Activation and movement of the tip in line with the canaliculus instantly clears away the obstruction. A probe is passed through the nasolacrimal duct to complete the operation.

Surgical Technique

1. Touch an activated 300-μm Fugo blade tip, set at medium energy and high power, to the supposed or known site of the punctum (Fig. 8.2).

2. Touch the tip vertically toward the first vertical section of the canaliculus to a penetration depth of only 0.5 mm.

3. Insert a lacrimal probe to determine whether it will negotiate through all of the canaliculus and the nasolacrimal duct. If it does, then pass thicker probes through the canaliculus and the nasolacrimal duct.

4. If the newly formed punctum looks reasonably good, nothing remains to be done. The size of the punctum can be increased with the Fugo blade.

Postoperative Management

Prescribe local steroid–antibiotic drops for five to six times a day and steroid–antibiotic ointment at bedtime. Advise the patient to carry out this regimen for 2 weeks.

Treatment of Canaliculus Closure

Opening the Vertical Portion of the Canaliculus

The vertical portion of the canaliculus is about 2 mm long and joins the horizontal canaliculus at a right angle called the "ampulla." When this part of the canaliculus in involved in scar formation, it is opened in the same way that the punctum is opened.

TECHNIQUE

Anesthesia

Infiltrate lidocaine 2% near the lid margin and use surface anesthesia.

Surgical Technique

1. Only the activated tip has to go deeper than a depth of 2 mm. Be very careful not to go through the wall of the canaliculus at the ampulla. Introduce the unactivated tip into the canaliculus, until it can go no further. Activate it without pressing it. This removes about 0.2 mm of the obstruction. Remove the tip and introduce a probe to see whether the desired depth has been achieved. If it has not, repeat the process until the ampulla is reached. The proof that you have achieved the goal is that the probe can be turned at a right angle and passed into the horizontal segment.

Opening the Horizontal Portion of the Canaliculus

The horizontal canaliculus is about 8 mm long. It usually joins the vertical canaliculus to form the common canaliculus, which immediately enters the nasolacrimal sac through the valve of Rosenmüller (a flap of mucosa to prevent reflux).

A canaliculus can close up as a result of any pathologic condition that produces raw areas on the canalicular wall, which may cause narrowing or obliteration of the lumen. The obliterated length and position varies. Canalicular obstruction can be caused by chlamydial infections (trachoma); viruses such as chickenpox and herpes simplex; bacterial diseases of the lids; or cicatrizing diseases such as ocular pemphigoid. Local medications and radiation can also cause canalicular obstruction, but most canalicular obstructions are idiopathic.

Patients with this condition suffer from intractable epiphora—a condition that is fairly common but often resistant to treatment. A forceful attempt to open the canaliculus with a lacrimal probe at best fails or at worst further damages the canaliculus. What is required is a clean removal of the obstructing epithelial or scar tissue without tearing or puncturing the canaliculus. This can be successfully achieved using the Fugo blade.

TECHNIQUE

Anesthesia

Infiltrate lidocaine 2% near the medial canaliculus.

Surgical Technique

1. Verify the obstruction site with a thin lacrimal probe. Then insert increasing sizes of lacrimal probes up to the locus of the obstruction. The idea is to make it easy for the fairly flexible Fugo blade tip to traverse the distance up to the obstruction with the least resistance and without bending.

2. Insert a 300-μm straight Fugo blade tip. It has a 200-μm sleeve of nonstick material, which gives the tip a total width of 0.7 mm. About 0.25 mm of the tip is bare. The sleeve ends abruptly and is flat at the end. The 300-μm filament is also flat at the end.

3. To reach the site of the obstruction, first pass the 300-μm tip vertically through the first part of the canaliculus and then turn nearly vertically to go through the canaliculus proper. (For right-handed surgeons, tackling the right canaliculus is easier than entering the left one. The opposite is true for the left-handed surgeons.) Stretch the lid straight to make the tip entry easier. The thick cable attached to the Fugo blade handle is rather heavy for the delicate work to be performed; drape the cable over your shoulder to get it out of the way and reduce the drag on the cable.

4. Push the Fugo blade tip up to the obstruction site. It is important at this stage that the stretching and straightening of the canaliculus and the ablating tip and the handle of the instrument are correctly

aligned because the tip will be activated and pushed simultaneously. Set the tip at medium power at high energy. The tip goes through the obstruction in a fraction of a second; push it all the way in until it strikes the bone.

5. Insert lacrimal probes of increasing sizes to ensure that the canaliculus is open and well dilated. Then pass a probe through the nasolacrimal duct, pressing through any obstruction that may be present. This procedure works if the canalicular wall is intact. As the tip ablates the obstructing tissue, the nonstick sleeve keeps the canalicular wall away, thus preventing perforation of the duct. Sometimes, as a result of pathology, previous failed attempts, or both, the canalicular walls may become an inseparable part of the scar tissue. In such cases, making or opening the canaliculus can be a guessing game, but usually in this cases a track will form through which a lacrimal probe can be passed, making the operation likely to be a success.

A successfully opened canaliculus may close again. It may happen days, weeks, or months after surgery, but it can be reopened with little or no problem.

Summary

Canalicular blockage is a common condition. A closed canaliculus is a great concern for the patient because of the continued tearing, and it is a difficult condition for the surgeon. A forceful mechanical attempt to open a recalcitrant canaliculus can only aggravate the condition. But we have successfully treated over 100 cases of canalicular blockage with Fugo blade.

Suggested Reading

Nasolacrimal duct, obstruction. Accessed January 3, 2010, at http://emedicine.medscape.com/article/1210141-overview.

Nasolacrimal duct, congenital anomalies. Accessed January 3, 2010, at http://emedicine.medscape.com/article/1210252-overview.

Failed Dacryocystorhinostomy

SUNITA MOHAN,
VIJETA DHIMAN,
HARISH K. BISHT,
SARAN K. SATSANGI

Obstruction of the nasolacrimal duct results in disrupted outflow of tears, a condition commonly known as "epiphora." Epiphora remains one of the most bothersome complications of lacrimal system obstruction and has social implications. In 1904, French ophthalmologist Adeo Toti introduced an operation that he called "dacryocystorhinostomy" for the treatment of obstructive epiphora. He proposed that after creating an external approach to the lacrimal sac, its portion near the canaliculi should be preserved and absorbed into the nose by creating a window in the lateral wall of the nose.

Toti's technique was modified by other surgeons. External dacryocystorhinostomy is now the most popular operation performed to treat nasolacrimal duct obstruction and the standard by which other treatment methods can be measured and compared.

The success rate of external dacryocystorhinostomy (DCR) has been reported between 80% and 99%, depending on the surgeon's experience. Primary DCR failure is commonly due to scarring at the rhinostomy site. Various other methods to relieve the obstruction of the nasolacrimal duct have been adopted. These include endoscopic DCR, endoscopic laser nasal DCR, dacryocystoplasty, and endoscopic radiofrequency–assisted DCR.

Numerous modifications in various surgical steps of the original DCR operation have been introduced over the years for a better surgical outcome, without altering the basic concept.

We present a new intervention using the Fugo blade under B-scan guidance in DCR that failed because of fibrous tissue at the osteotomy site. The objective of our study was to determine the success rate of this technique in management of a failed DCR.

TECHNIQUE

This prospective study was conducted at Sarojini Naidu Medical College, Agra, India, from November 2006 through February 2008. A total of 11 patients who had failed DCRs were recruited—all from the outpatient department. The inclusion criteria were epiphora and a history of a previous DCR surgery. All patients recruited for the surgery were evaluated. Complete ophthalmic examination was performed, including determination of visual acuity, corneal opacities or ulceration, and other ocular comorbidity. Patients were then assessed with a lacrimal sac regurgitation test, syringing, probing, and nasal examination.

B-scanning of the sac area was performed to look for possible causes of obstruction. Patients who exhibited fibrous tissue at the osteotomy site as detected on B-scan were included in the study. All patients were also systemically evaluated for diabetes mellitus and hypertension (Figs. 9.1–9.3).

None of the patients was subjected to Schirmer's test, Jones test, or dacryocystography because simple regurgitation, syringing, and probing provided ample proof of the level of blockage in the lacrimal system. Written informed consent was obtained from all patients.

Anesthesia

All operations were performed under local anesthesia. Nasal packing was done with gauze soaked in 4% Xylocaine (lidocaine) and 1 in 100,000 adrenaline

9

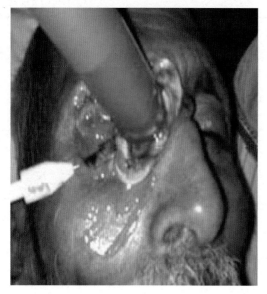

Figure 9.1. The Fugo probe tip inserted though the lower puncta and B-scan probe applied to the sac area.

Figure 9.3. The Fugo tip introduced into the sac area (*long arrow*) and cutting fibrous tissue (*short arrow*).

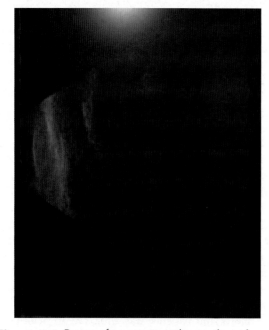

Figure 9.2. B-scan of an anastomotic area (*arrow*) showing fibrous tissue.

Surgical Technique

1. Insert the Fugo plasma blade into the lower punctum, lower canaliculus, and then into the sac anastomosis under B-scan guidance.

2. Excise the resistance encountered using the plasma blade.

3. Visualize endoscopically and resect any scar tissue.

Postoperative Management

The nasal pack was removed postoperatively. Patients were prescribed gatifloxacin (Zymar) eye drops three times daily for 2 weeks and oral ciprofloxacin 500 mg twice daily for 2 weeks and diclofenac 25 mg twice daily for 1 week.

Follow-up was done on the first and second postoperative days and 10 days, 1 month, and 6 months after the surgery. Syringing was done on the 10th postoperative day to assess the patency of the lacrimal system. A successful outcome was defined as resolution of symptoms such as epiphora and discharge and a patent lacrimal system on irrigation.

(epinephrine). Proper packing of the nasal cavity helped to anesthetize the mucosa, achieving good hemostasis. The area surrounding the lacrimal sac was infiltrated with 2% lidocaine with 1 in 100,000 epinephrine. About 4 to 5 ml of lidocaine was enough for successful anesthesia of the area.

Table 9.1. Age Distribution of Patients Treated for Failed Dacryocystorhinostomy

Age (yr)	No. (%)
31–40	3 (27.3)
41–50	4 (36.4)
51–60	4 (36.4)
Total	11 (100)

Note: Percentages do not add to 100 because of rounding.

Table 9.2. Complications during Surgery

Complication	No. (%)
Bleeding from nasal mucosa	1 (9.1)
Bleeding from nasal bone	1 (9.1)
Nasal mucosal tearing	0
None	9 (81.8)
Total	11 (100)

Summary

Eleven patients underwent intervention for failed DCR with this Fugo blade technique. Most patients were between 41 and 60 years of age (72.7%) (Table 9.1).

The study participants were predominantly female (72.2%). Women have significantly smaller dimensions in the lower nasolacrimal fossa and middle nasolacrimal duct. Hormonal changes that bring about a generalized de-epithelization in the body may cause the same within the lacrimal sac and duct. An already narrow lacrimal fossa in women predisposes them to obstruction by sloughed off debris. In addition, the injudicious use of cheap or adulterated eye cosmetics applied to the wrong side of the eyelashes can also play important role in obstruction of the nasolacrimal system.

All patients were operated on under local anesthesia. Selection of proper anesthesia is vital for the success of a procedure. The advantages of local anesthesia are that it is relatively cheap and safe, and when properly administered it is as effective as general anesthesia.

During surgery, some patients experienced bleeding from the nasal mucosa, bleeding from nasal bone, or both. Nasal mucosal tearing was seen in none. Surgery was uneventful in 10 patients (81.8%) (Table 9.2). No complications such as bleeding from the nose, wound infection, or cellulitis were seen in the immediate postoperative period. The overall success rate was 91% after an average follow-up of 6 months. Only 1 patient continued to have troublesome epiphora and required further surgery. The cause of failure in this case was small osteotomy size.

Summary

Using the Fugo plasma blade to repair a failed DCR had several advantages. Pain and hemorrhaging were minimal, postoperative facial swelling and scarring were absent, and symptoms resolved rapidly after surgery. This is the first study to use the Fugo plasma blade to treat a failed DCR. No incision, no sutures, no pain, no blood, and a nearly 100% success rate are all factors likely to make the Fugo blade the choice of many surgeons in the future to manage cases of failed DCR.

Suggested Reading

McGrath D. Fugo blade effective tool for multiple surgical applications. *Eurotimes.* 2008;13(6):43.

Singh D. Peep-hole surgery for dacryocystitis. *Trop Ophthalmol.* 2002;2:11–12.

10 Entropion of the Upper Eyelid

DALJIT SINGH and
SEEMA K. SINGH

T rachoma is one of the most common causes of upper eyelid entropion and trichiasis. The corneal lesions result either as sequelae of eyelid deformity or from dryness of the eye resulting from partial to total destruction of secretory elements of the conjunctiva and keratinization of the epithelium.

Entropion and trichiasis cause eye irritation because the affected eyelid rubs against the cornea and conjunctiva. Surgical correction of the lid deformity is important for relief of irritation and to avoid further damage to the eye.

Entropion results from cicatricial contraction of the tarsal conjunctiva, which pulls the intermarginal strip up and in, rounding off the sharp inner edge. This in turn pulls on the skin, and the lashes become misdirected, turning inward. The change in the direction of the lashes begins in the hindmost row first. As the severity of the contraction increases, more rows of the cilia turn inward.

The correction of entropion is best done from the conjunctival side, because the incision goes through the scar tissue of the conjunctiva and the nearest part of the tarsal plate. The key operation for entropion of the upper lid is the "inversio tarsi"; this procedure has various modifications of the conjunctival approach to entropion correction. The surgery involves the rotation of the distal (lash-bearing) end of the tarsal plate by undermining it with the wedge of the proximal (toward the fornix) end of the tarsal plate and securing it in place by suturing proximal tarsal plate to the undersurface of the skin bearing the lashes.

TECHNIQUE

Anesthesia

Use topical anesthesia for surface anesthesia for the conjunctiva, and infiltrate the lid with proparacaine 1%, which provides good anesthesia. Balloon the lid with anesthetic and apply pressure for a few minutes.

Surgical Technique

1. Pass a thick nylon suture close to the upper lid margin and hold it with an artery forceps. The suture acts as a kind of "leash" during the surgery.

2. Evert the lid over a Desmarre lid retractor. The conjunctival side of the lid is visible from end to end. The subtarsal sulcus is visible about 1.5 to 2 mm behind the root of the cilia. Its distance from the cilia is closer in the middle, but usually increases toward the two ends (Fig. 10.1).

3. Use a Fugo blade with a 100-μm tip (used for capsulotomy) at high energy settings. Make an incision at the subtarsal sulcus from end to end. The first pass should be about half depth of the tarsal plate. Press the lid retractor upward to keep the tarsal plate stretched. Cut the tarsal plate deeper first in the middle and then on the sides.

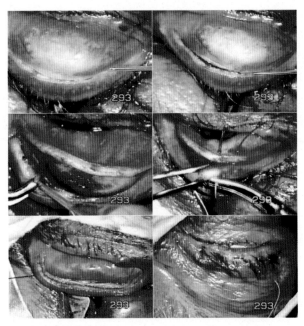

Figure 10.1. The lid is everted using a Desmarre rectractor. Incision is made with the Fugo blade with a 100-μm tip at the subtarsal sulcus and deepened until the tarsal plate is cut. Undermining of the tarsal plate is done on both sides with a 600-μm Fugo blade tip. The cut edges are sutured so that the lid margin bearing the cilia rotates forward.

As you cut the middle part of the plate to full depth, the pressure of the lid spatula separates the cut edges. Then extend the incision on both sides. The lid spatula is the sheet anchor for presenting the stretched tarsal plate for incision and for hemostasis when a lid vessel is cut. You can minimize or even avoid bleeding if you carry out the deepest part of the incision very slowly, so that you do not injure any large blood vessel passing through the orbicularis muscle. Although the pressure of the lid spatula controls the leakage of blood, use a 600-μm Fugo blade tip at the medium power setting to stop bleeding.

4. Undermine the entire cut edges of the tarsal plate to separate it from the orbicularis muscle on both sides for about 2 mm, using the same 600-μm tip. The Fugo blade tip maintains hemostasis at the same time. Take care not to damage the roots of the eyelashes.

5. Suture with a 5-0 absorbable polyglactin suture. Begin at the lateral edge from the skin surface of the lid. Pass the needle through the skin along the lashes so that the tip emerges from under the distal cut edge of the tarsal plate. On the proximal side, make it to traverse from the anterior to the posterior surface like a whip. Then make the suture traverse back the same way, starting about 3 mm away, avoiding any picking of the orbicularis muscle. Repeat the same steps in a key pattern, until the whole lid margin is covered. Then stretch and tighten the suture between two needle holders, and make it take a bite of the skin to reach the first entry point, where you should tie it.

Postoperative Management

Apply a dressing for 4 to 5 hours. Prescribe an antibiotic ointment to be used twice a day for 3 weeks. The sutures do not need to be removed; internal sutures are absorbed, and exposed sutures fall off in a couple of weeks.

Suggested Reading

Duke-Elder W. System of ophthalmology, vol. 8. London: Kimpton, 1965.

Kettesy A. Genesis and operation of cicatricial (trachomatous) entropion of the upper lid. *Br J Ophthalmol.* 1948;32:419–423.

Mukherjee PK, Jain PC. Entropion operation of upper lid in trachoma—a modification of "inversio tarsi" operation. *Indian J. Ophthalmol.* 1969;17:99–102.

Shukla BR. Surgical consideration in trachoma cases in India. *J All-India Ophthalmol Soc.* 1964;12:82–84.

Part B
The Conjunctiva

11 | Limbal Nevus DALJIT SINGH

y colleagues and I have successfully used the Fugo blade to remove a large nevus along the limbus of a 2-year-old patient.

TECHNIQUE

Anesthesia

Administer general anesthesia.

Surgical Technique

1. At 2 mm away from the nevus, puncture the conjunctiva with a 100-μm Fugo blade. Through this opening, introduce a 30-gauge cannula and inject saline to balloon the conjunctiva and lift it from the surface of the sclera. Using a cannula instead of a needle prevents subconjunctival bleeding (Fig. 11.1).

2. Make an incision in the ballooned conjunctiva with the same Fugo blade tip about 1 mm from the edge of the lesion. If the conjunctiva flattens out before the incision can be completed, lift it away from the sclera with a forceps and then cut. Do not touch the sclera.

3. Touch any blood vessel coursing toward the lesion seen in the subconjunctival tissues with a 600-μm Fugo blade tip set at low energy.

4. Life the nevus and dissect it toward the limbus with a 100-μm Fugo blade tip until the limbus comes in to view. Once again, touch any visible blood vessel with a 600-μm tip set at low energy.

5. Use corneal scissors to excise the conjunctiva carrying the nevus, right up to the cornea. The nevus can be removed completely with this technique. A small portion of pigment might still be visible.

6. To make certain that no nevus tissue is left, momentarily touch the suspected area of the limbus with the 600-μm tip.

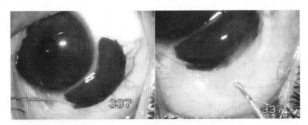
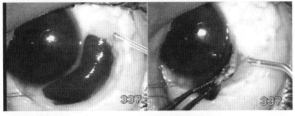
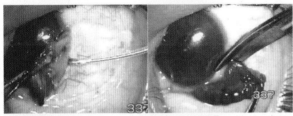
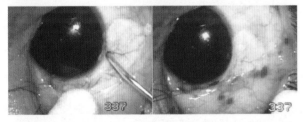

7. Undermine the incised conjunctiva with scissors. Bring the conjunctiva forward and suture it to the sclera. Some bare sclera is inevitable at the end of the surgery, but it will be covered up during the postoperative period.

Summary

A limbal nevus can be removed using forceps, scissors, and bipolar cautery, but at the risk of excessive tissue trauma. Excision of a nevus using the Fugo blade can be done with finesse, precision, and little or no tissue trauma.

Suggested Reading

Kellan R, Fugo RJ. Device increases safety, efficiency of cataract surgery. *Ophthalmol Times.* 2000;25:7–9.

Roy FH. Course for Fugo blade is enlightening, surgeon says. *Ocular Surg News.* 2001;19:35–38.

Figure 11.1. Excision of a large limbal nevus. The conjunctiva is ballooned and incised with a 100-μm tip around the lesion. The 600-μm tip ablates the underlying blood vessels. The nevus-carrying conjunctiva is excised with the scissors. The remnant of the nevus is ablated with the 600-μm tip. The undermined conjunctiva is brought forward and sutured to the sclera, leaving some bare sclera.

12 Limbal Nodule DALJIT SINGH

An unusual-looking nodule at the limbus should always lead you to suspect a malignancy, and it must be removed in toto. It is important to achieve clean margins when removing these nodules, so as not to leave any tissue that might prove malignant later on. A nodule may have excessive vascularity, which must be addressed during excision. Bipolar cautery or heat cautery can serve this purpose, but these often cause unnecessary trauma to the tissues. The following cases illustrate how the Fugo blade can be used in removing limbal nodules.

CASE STUDIES

Case 1

A 60-year-old farmer had noticed the formation and growth of a "white thing" at the limbus for over 6 months. A 5-mm hard white lesion sitting astride the lateral limbus appeared heavily vascularized.

TECHNIQUE

Anesthesia

Make a hole was made in the conjunctiva with a 100-μm Fugo blade tip. Administer lignocaine 2% through a cannula to inflate it around the lesion.

Surgical Technique

1. Use a hockey-stick knife to separate the nodule from the corneal side (ours succeeded only partially).

2. Incise the conjunctiva all around the lesion with a 300-μm Fugo blade tip at low energy and medium power setting.

3. Push the lesion and cut toward the limbus with the same tip. Remove only the top layers.

4. Lift the remaining tissue over the surface of the sclera with a forceps and perform ablation until the field became reasonably clean (Fig. 12.1).

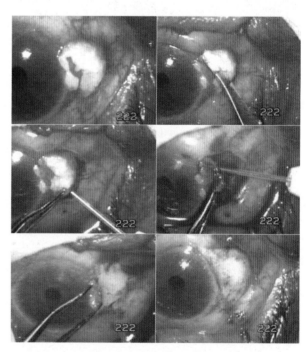

Figure 12.1. A hard nodule at the limbus. The hockey-stick knife was ineffective. The nodule is dissected free of the underlying tissues with a 300-μm Fugo blade tip, and the base of the nodule is polished clean with a 600-μm Fugo blade tip.

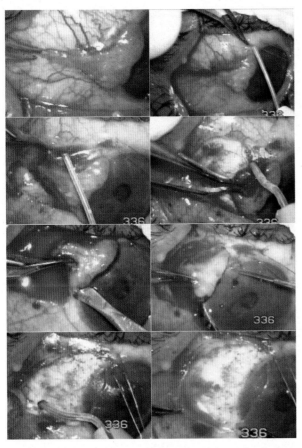

Figure 12.2. A fleshy vascularized mass is at the limbus. The mass is lifted with lidocaine after making a conjunctival hole with 100-μm Fugo blade tip. The fornix side is cut, lifted, and dissected toward the limbus. Next the limbal side is lifted and the whole mass is removed. The based is cleaned and polished with the 600-μm Fugo blade tip.

5. Remove the nodular tissue remaining on the cornea with a fine forceps. Then use a 600-μm Fugo blade tip a medium power and energy to clear and polish the cornea, limbus, and exposed sclera. Rub the activated tip under a stream of saline, removing the remaining lesion without excessive loss of healthy tissue.

6. Leave the sclera bare for coverage by the conjunctiva in the postoperative period.

Postoperative Management

Prescribe mitomycin 0.02% for instillation seven to eight times a day for a period of 7 days, along with antibiotic–steroid ointment three times a day. In our case, the histologic examination report received after 1 week was negative for malignancy, and the patient had an uneventful recovery.

Case 2

A 57-year-old truck driver presented with a fleshy vascularized nodule on the medial side of the cornea. The appearance of the nodule was unusual, almost the reverse of a commonly seen pterygium with the fleshy base situated toward the cornea and the apex toward the medial canthus. The nodule was removed in a manner similar to that used in Case 1 (Fig. 12.2). The histologic examination report received after 1 week was negative for malignancy. This patient, too, had an uneventful recovery.

Summary

Use of the Fugo blade to remove unusual limbal lesions has one great advantage: the ability to remove the finest visible remains of pathologic tissue with greater accuracy and with minimal damage to normal tissue.

Suggested Reading

Kellan R, Fugo RJ. Device increases safety, efficiency of cataract surgery. *Ophthalmol Times*. 2000;25:7–9.

Roy FH. Course for Fugo blade is enlightening, surgeon says. *Ocular Surg News*. 2001;19:3538.

13 Carcinoma In Situ of the Conjuctiva DALJIT SINGH

Carcinoma in situ represents the malignant end of the spectrum of conjunctival dysplasias. The lesion may undergo spontaneous regression. It may start anywhere in the conjunctiva and cornea, but often starts at the limbus as an opaque, white, shiny, fleshy mass arising from the epithelium of the conjunctiva. It may present as a leukoplakia, a papilloma, or a complication of pterygium or pinguecula. The mass is similar to squamous epithelial lesions found elsewhere in the mucous membrane.

The basal membrane of the epithelium remains intact, and the subepithelial tissue is not invaded. Only infrequently does the lesion becomes invasive. Features include acanthosis, total loss of normal cellular maturation and cytologic atypia affecting the full thickness of the epithelium large and elongated tumor cells with the long axis of the cells oriented perpendicular to the basal lamina, and parakeratosis and mitotic activity in all layers.

Between 1999 and the present my colleagues and I have operated on three cases of carcinoma in situ, using the ablative properties of the Fugo blade to eradicate the last vestiges of diseased tissue. In one of these cases, the surgery had to be repeated.

CASE STUDY

The patient was 67 years of age. The lesion involved most of the limbus and the adjoining conjunctiva and cornea. The lower medial, upper medial, and lateral areas were particularly involved.

TECHNIQUE

Anesthesia

Administer surface anesthesia. Then puncture the conjunctiva with a 100-μm Fugo blade tip and inject 2% lignocaine with epinephrine through it using a blunt cannula to avoid possible subconjunctival hemorrhage from a needle prick. Balloon the conjunctiva with anesthetic fluid.

Surgical Technique

1. Incise the conjunctiva 0.5 mm beyond the visible limit of the pathologic area using a 100-μm tip, to ensure that the incision does not go deeper than the conjunctiva. Lift the conjunctiva and also incise the subconjunctival tissue carrying the blood vessels. Ablating the blood vessels in the path of the incision ensures that no malignant cells are carried away. Lift the conjunctiva toward the limbus.

2. Life the visible corneal presence of the lesion with a hockey-stick knife. After removing the diseased tissue, the base is ready to be cleaned.

3. Smooth and clean the base using a 600-μm Fugo blade tip like an eraser. Set the energy at medium power and intensity. Apply the blade under a continuous saline stream, so that ablation and the clearing process are under greater control. Glide the activated tip over the surface of the sclera, the

limbus, and the cornea, without pressing. Continue the process until a satisfactory surface appearance is achieved.

4. Undermine the conjunctiva around the cut edge and bring it forward and suture it to the sclera, leaving the perilimbal area bare.

5. Apply a bandage contact lens to reduce postoperative pain as well as to improve the efficacy of the local antimitotic drops (Figs. 13.1–13.3).

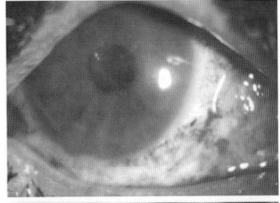

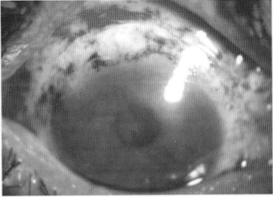

Figure 13.2. The appearance of the eye 4 days after surgery. The bandage contact lens is visible.

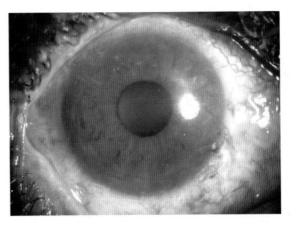

Figure 13.3. The same patient 1.5 years after surgery. The appearance of the eye is satisfactory.

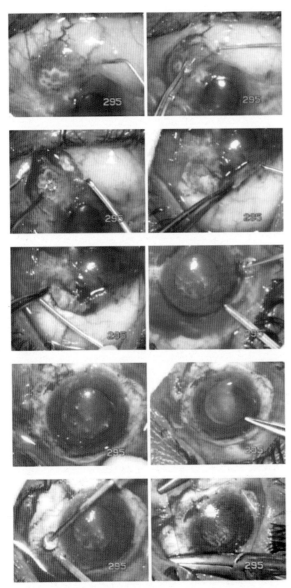

Figure 13.1. The conjunctiva is ballooned with local anesthetic. Incision is made with a 100-μm Fugo blade in the conjunctiva and excision is carried toward the limbus. Remaining tissue is ablated with a 600-μm Fugo blade tip under a stream of saline. The conjunctiva is brought forward and sutured some distance from the limbus. A bandage contact lens is applied.

Postoperative Management

Instruct the patient to instill local mitomycin drops 0.04% seven to eight times a day. These drops should be kept in a refrigerator and prepared fresh every third day. Continue the mitomycin treatment for 15 days. Concurrently, use local antibiotic–steroid ointment twice a day.

In our case, the histology report assured the patient and the surgeon of a good prognosis. However, regular critical examination of the eye is important to guard against recurrence. Any recurrence should be treated in the same manner.

Summary

Using the Fugo blade to manage carcinoma in situ offers some advantages over the use of traditional instruments such as forceps, scissors, and cautery.

Tissue removal by ablation with the Fugo blade rather than raw cutting ensures that no pathologic cells escape via the blood vessels or the lymphatics. Furthermore, the finest remnants of the tumor on the sclera, limbus, and cornea are removed with greater confidence.

Suggested Reading

Kellan R, Fugo RJ. Device increases safety, efficiency of cataract surgery. *Ophthalmol Times*. 2000;25:7–9.

Roy FH. Course for Fugo blade is enlightening, surgeon says. *Ocular Surg News*. 2001;19:35–38.

Bitot's Spots DALJIT SINGH

Bitot's spots are considered a sign of past or present vitamin A deficiency; however, some patients do not respond to vitamin therapy. Patients with Bitot's spots appear with disfigured conjunctiva, and some may have night blindness and punctate keratopathy. Histologically, keratinization with granular cells appears with irregular maturation, inflammatory infiltration of the conjunctival substantia propria, and loss of goblet cells. Prominent Bitot's spots may represent massive accumulations of gram-positive bacilli and keratin debris.

For patients who are nonresponsive to vitamin A therapy, the available treatment for Bitot's spots is excision of the defective conjunctiva. We have used the Fugo blade to remove these unsightly conjunctival spots.

CASE STUDIES

Case 1

The patient was a 19-year-old army recruit who was rejected because of the bilateral presence of Bitot's spots.

TECHNIQUE

Anesthesia

Administer surface anesthesia. Then puncture the conjunctiva with a 100-μm Fugo blade tip close to the edge of the incision, and inject 2% lignocaine through it using a thin cannula to avoid possible subconjunctival hemorrhage from a needle prick. Balloon the conjunctiva with anesthetic fluid.

Surgical Technique

Sweep a 600-μm Fugo blade tip at the lowest energy setting over the surface of the lesion from one edge to the other until the conjunctiva appeared to be reasonably clear of the spot. Perform this in both eyes at the same setting (Fig. 14.1).

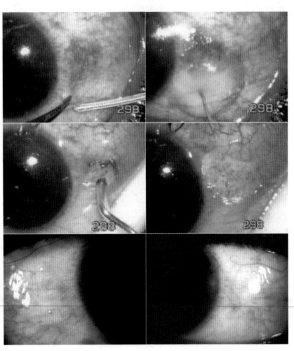

Figure 14.1. The conjunctiva is punctured close to the edge of lesion with a 100-μm tip. Lignocaine is injected through this hole to raise the conjunctiva. A 600-μm Fugo blade tip is swept over the lesion. **Bottom:** The two eyes 10 days after treatment.

Postoperative Management

Do not apply a dressing. Prescribe antibiotic–steroid ointment to be used twice a day for 10 days. In our case, the eyes were clear enough for the recruit to join the military service.

Case 2

The patient in this case was a well-nourished 5-year-old boy in whom Bitot's spots had been seen since the age of 6 months, soon after he suffered a bout of severe diarrhea. His classmates at school often commented on the odd appearance of his eyes.

The patient was given general anesthesia for the procedure. The Bitot's spots were easily removed with the sweeping motion of the 600-μm Fugo blade tip over the conjunctiva. It took a couple of seconds to treat each eye. Steroid–antibiotic ointment was prescribed. Ten days after treatment, the conjunctiva looked normal (Fig. 14.2).

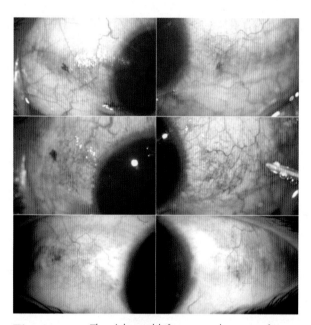

Figure 14.2. The right and left eyes at the start of surgery, at the end of surgery, and 10 days after surgery.

Summary

The Fugo blade is particularly effective in removing Bitot's spots and similar surface lesions with great ease.

Suggested Reading

Ahed MA, et al. Bitot's spots following hemicolectomy. *Eye* 2003;17:671–673.

Baker BM, Bender DA, eds. *Vitamins in medicine*, vol. 2, 4th ed. London: Heinemann, 1982; p. 222.

Emran N, Tjakrasudjatma S. Clinical characteristics of vitamin A responsive and nonresponsive Bitot's spots. *Am J Ophthalmol*. 1980;90:160–171.

Part C
Extraocular Muscles

Strabismus DALJIT SINGH and ARUN VERMA

Strabismus is a very common condition that often needs surgical treatment to make the eyes orthophoric, prevent amblyopia, and promote binocularity and stereopsis. In this surgery, the various rectus muscles are recessed or resected; the oblique muscles are mostly cut, not strengthened. The instruments used are very basic: forceps, scissors, and bipolar cautery. The sutures used are usually absorbable. Surgery is followed by continued oozing to frank bleeding. The tenon capsule is difficult to exactly define, cut, and keep and suture in place. The extraocular muscle is detached from the insertion for both recession and resection purposes. Perfect realignment of the detached muscle may not be obtained while suturing. Postoperative reaction and scarring of the operated area are common. Repeat surgery on the same muscle is quite difficult.

By virtue of its ability to ablate tissues bloodlessly, use of the Fugo blade as a cutting and ablating tool brings about a sea change in how surgery on extraocular muscles may be done in the future. This extraordinary facilitation has permitted us to improve the surgical technique, reduce surgery time, increase the accuracy of alignment, minimize postoperative problems, and rehabilitate the patient more quickly. The surgical management of recti and the oblique muscles is described below.

Block Removal/Recession of a Rectus Muscle

The philosophy of this new recession procedure is not to detach the muscle but to weaken it by removing a muscle block while leaving intact a thin strip of muscle on either side. It may be likened to a sutureless recession. The vascularity of muscle tissue close to the insertion is not touched, therefore no danger of anterior segment necrosis exists if more than one muscle is addressed. The insertion can be cut selectively to reduce hypertropia or hypotropia. Because misalignment of the muscle is out of the question, the technique can be safely applied in cases of symptomatic phorias.

TECHNIQUE

Anesthesia

Most strabismus surgery is in pediatric patients, so general anesthesia is the normal choice. Under anesthesia,

15

the eyeball may roll up and rotate, but this action will not prevent accurate positioning of the extraocular muscle.

Surgical Technique

1. Fixing the eyeball: Pass a suture through the episclera close to the limbus and weight it to expose the surgical area. We use an 80-μm vanadium steel suture for this purpose.

2. Use a Lim forceps to nudge the edge of the muscle to determine its position. As the muscle edge engages the forceps, the eyeball rotates.

3. Make the conjunctival-tenon incision over the muscle as far away from the limbus as possible. On the nasal side, make the incision under the plica semilunaris, so that in the end the incision line is buried. Not dissecting the conjunctiva from the limbal side and not making large conjunctival flaps helps to prevent unnecessary injury to the tenon capsule and damage to the subconjunctival lymphatics and consequent scarring. Use a 100-μm Fugo blade tip at the lowest energy settings. Life the conjunctiva as it is being incised. The incision deepens imperceptibly with the incision of tenon capsule. Life the tenon capsule every time the incision is deepened. As the thickness of the tenon capsule is crossed, you will encounter very loose tenon connective tissue under which the muscle belly or tendon is clearly visible. The tenon capsule is very thick in children and needs bloodless ablation layer by layer until the muscle fibers become visible. Extend the incision up and down to reach the muscle edges. Once the edges have been defined, insert a muscle hook underneath it. Hold the tenon capsule with a forceps at the edge of the muscle and strip the capsule toward the fornix. Treat the other edge of the muscle in the same way. Once you strip the tenon capsule, it becomes easy to insert the second muscle hook and stretch the muscle between the two hooks. Hold any remnant of the capsule in the surgical field with a fine forceps and remove it with the Fugo blade. The whole process is bloodless (Fig. 15.1).

4. Next, remove a block of the muscle to weaken it. The effect of this step is similar to the recession of the muscle. Depending on the weakening that is to be achieved, choose the proximal point on the muscle and bring the proximal muscle hook under it. Use the activated Fugo blade tip to make two longitudinal full-thickness cuts on the muscle over the muscle hook. Make each cut about

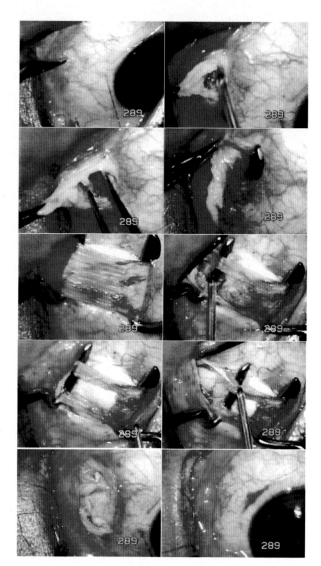

Figure 15.1. Medical rectus weakening. The forceps tip is used to find the edge of the muscle. The Fugo blade makes incisions through the conjunctiva and tenon capsule. The exposed muscle is stretched between muscle hooks. A block of muscle is removed, followed by marginal tenotomy of the remaining muscle strips. The tenon capsule and conjunctiva are sutured in layers.

1 mm from the edge of the muscle. Never make the incision without a metallic support underneath, otherwise the sclera will be incised instantly. Advance the incisions toward the insertion over a metal spatula (the lens spatula). Stop the incisions short of the insertion, so that the blood vessel–bearing distal portion of the muscle is left untouched for about 1.5 mm. Now take the proximal muscle hook back again under the initial incisions. Cut the muscle vertically between the two incisions, over the muscle hook. The cut muscle block now hangs free from the insertion

side. Lift it with a utility forceps and cut with Fugo blade about 1.5 mm from the insertion. At this point an approximately 1.5-mm strip of the intact muscle exists at insertion, from which a 1-mm strip along either edge stretches to the proximal part of the muscle. There is a rectangular empty area from which the block of muscle has been removed. Depending on the requirements of the case, further weaken the muscle by performing marginal tenotomy on the muscle strips that are left after block removal. The whole process is essentially bloodless and unaccompanied by tissue charring. The occasional bleeder can be touched with a 600-μm Fugo blade tip at the lowest setting. To improve concomitant hypertropia or hypotropia, cut the muscle strip along one edge, so that the eyeball gets more support toward the uncut side.

5. Bring the tenon capsule and conjunctiva together in layers. The cut edges of the tenon capsule are easy to pick. We use 40-μm vanadium steel sutures for this purpose because they are nonmagnetic, cause no inflammation, and need no removal. The conjunctival sutures do not irritate and will eventually fall off. Absorbable sutures are also acceptable.

Postoperative Management

The postoperative period is usually uneventful. No postoperative edema results after block removal/ recession.

Block Removal plus Plication/Resection

Surgical steps for block removal plus plication/resection are the same with regard to exposing muscle weakening. The muscle is stripped of the tenon capsule and stretched between the two muscle hooks (Fig. 15.2).

Surgical Technique

1. Pass an 80-μm vanadium steel suture through the belly of the muscle at the desired distance from the insertion. Pass the suture twice and then fasten it.

2. Block removal of the muscle is the next step. Keep the Fugo blade away from the knot, as touching the steel suture with the activated Fugo blade can weaken and even break the suture.

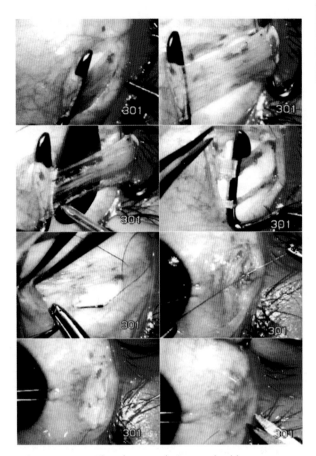

Figure 15.2. After the muscle is stretched between two muscle hooks, an anchoring 80-μm steel suture is passed through the belly of the muscle. Incisions are made to remove a block of the muscle and to leave thin strips along the two edges. The anchoring suture is passed through the insertion and tied. Notice the presence of a spatula beneath the muscle when the strips are being created with the Fugo blade.

3. Loose the eyeball-fixating suture. Pass the advancement suture through the episclera at the insertion of the muscle. Tie the suture in a reef knot and cut close to the knot. The suture should not project forward or it will cause severe irritation. Although our preference is for steel sutures, an absorbable suture can be used.

4. Suture the tenon capsule and the conjunctiva in layers.

Postoperative Management

Patients feel discomfort for a few hours after plication/advancement because the muscle has been stretched.

15

Surgery on the Vertical Muscles

The surgery of the vertical muscles is just the same as in the case of the horizontal muscles. The Fugo blade technique of block removal completely avoids dealing with the sclera.

Surgery on the Inferior Oblique Muscle

Overaction of the inferior oblique muscle is frequently responsible for hypertropia. The treatment is myomectomy of the inferior oblique muscle. In the usual approach, muscle body is exposed from either the skin side or the conjunctival side, held between artery forceps, and cut. This is easier said than done. Bleeding from cutting the conjunctiva and tenon capsule makes the surgery cumbersome. Using the Fugo blade makes the surgery bloodless and clean (Fig.15.3).

TECHNIQUE

Surgical Technique

1. Reveal the edge of the inferior rectus by nudging with a forceps about 10 to 12 mm from the limbus. The inferior oblique muscle passes underneath this muscle horizontally near the equator of the eye.
2. To approach the belly of the inferior oblique muscle, make an incision in the conjunctiva with the Fugo blade about 8 to 10 mm temporal to the lateral edge of the inferior rectus and about 12 to 15 mm from the limbus. Then lift and cut the tenon capsule until the sclera becomes visible.
3. Use a stout forceps to move the sclera over to reach and hold the belly of the inferior oblique muscle and pull it out in the incision line. The tenon capsule covering of the muscle is quite thick. Pass the Fugo blade underneath the muscle and the tenon capsule. Then pass a muscle hook through the track made by the Fugo blade, followed by a second muscle hook. Stretch the inferior oblique muscle between the two hooks.
4. No artery forceps is used to clamp the muscle. Incise the highly vascular and muscular belly

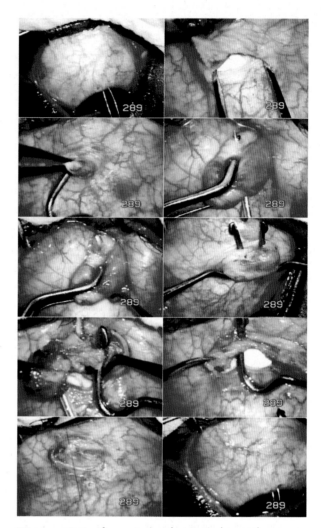

Figure 15.3. After exposing the surgical area, the conjunctiva and tenon capsule are cut with the Fugo blade to expose the sclera. The inferior oblique muscle is pulled out and a Fugo blade track is made under the muscle through the tenon capsule to make room for the muscle hooks. The stretched muscle is attenuated with the Fugo blade. The incision is closed in layers.

gradually with a 300-μm or 600-μm Fugo blade tip at low energy settings. The muscle is ablated without bleeding. Some muscle fibers are left intact; create a gap by removing a 4- to 5-mm length of the muscle. Touch any bleeder with the 600-μm tip. Remove the muscle hooks.

5. Close the tenon capsule and conjunctiva separately with a couple of 40-μm vanadium steel sutures. Absorbable sutures can also be used for closing the incisions.

Surgery on the superior oblique muscle is similar. The muscle may best be located on the nasal side of the superior rectus muscle.

Repeated Surgery on Extraocular Muscle

Repeated surgery on any extraocular muscle is often difficult because of the presence of scar tissue in the operative field. Ordinarily, dissection is difficult—having to cut through scar tissue to define and operate on the muscle. Bleeding is another problem. The Fugo blade makes resurgery much easier.

Summary

The Fugo blade makes surgery on extraocular muscles bloodless and efficient. The surgical time spent on each muscle is about 7 to 8 minutes. The block removal technique provides a new kind of recession, and plication preserves muscle vascularity near the insertion, thereby abolishing the risk of anterior segment necrosis. Every extraocular muscle is easy to approach and operate. Phoria cases can be operated with greater confidence. Because the blood vessels are closed during Fugo blade incisions on the tenon capsule and the muscle, little postoperative reaction results and recovery is therefore quick. Keeping the incisions away from the limbus preserves the conjunctival lymphatics and minimizes tenon capsule scarring.

Suggested Reading

Singh D, Singh RSJ, Kaur H, et al. Plasma powered squint surgery with the Fugo blade. *Ann Ophthalmol.* 2003;35:12–14.

16 Cysticercus DALJIT SINGH

Cysticercus cellulosae, the larval form of the pork tapeworm *Taenia solium,* is the causative organism of cysticercosis. Humans are the intermediate hosts in this organism's life cycle. Cysticercus cellulosae may become encysted in various tissues, usually the eyes, central nervous system, and subcutaneous tissues. An immunologic reaction with fairly intense inflammatory signs and symptoms may be produced, and the surrounding structures may be compressed. This disorder is common in countries with people living in conditions of poor hygiene.

Ocular cysticercosis may be extra-ocular or intraocular. Depending on the location, different symptoms and signs arise. Cysticercosis of the subconjunctival or extraocular muscle presents as a painful, yellowish, nodular subconjunctival mass with surrounding conjunctival congestion. The tissue reaction creates a fibrous wall around the cyst, which becomes thicker over time.

Only the accessible subconjunctival or extraocular muscle cysticercus can be surgically removed. Because the cyst usually adheres to surrounding tissues, including the extraocular muscles, excision is difficult. And because the goal is to completely remove the parasite along with the cyst wall, bleeding and trauma to the tissues, including the extraocular muscle, are unavoidable. The extent of tissue trauma depends on the surgical tools used and the complexity of the case.

We have operated on four cases of cysticercus that were visible as subconjunctival swellings. Two case examples are described below.

CASE STUDIES

Case 1

The patient was a 10-year-old child who had increasing swelling and redness toward the medical canthus for over 2 weeks. The swelling was circumscribed and tender to the touch. The clinical diagnosis was cysticercus. Oral steroids were prescribed for 2 days before surgery.

TECHNIQUE

Anesthesia

The surgery was done under general anesthesia.

Surgical Technique

1. Use the Fugo blade capsulotomy tip at the lowest energy settings. Hold the conjunctiva over the most prominent part of the cyst with a forceps. Make a tiny exploratory incision close to the forceps. The conjunctiva separate without any resistance or bleeding.

2. Extend the incision cautiously into the cyst wall, up and down, going slightly deeper every time (Fig. 16.1) until the cyst eventually appears at the incision line. Very cautiously enlarge the incision further, until the cyst begins to extrude

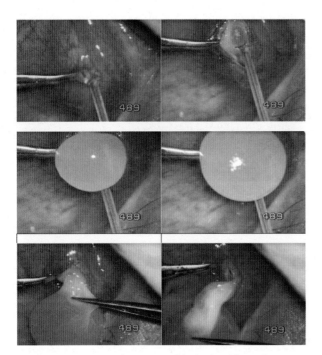

Figure 16.1. A 100-μm Fugo blade tip ablates the cyst wall, through which the cyst spontaneously extrudes. The final portion of the cyst containing the scolex is pulled out with a plain forceps.

spontaneously from the incision. Make no attempt to grasp the cyst at this stage. When most of the cyst is out, hold it at the scolex with a plane forceps and remove it completely. No sutures are needed.

As expected, our patient made a quick recovery. It could not be determined whether the cyst was connected with the extraocular muscle underneath. There was no way to know, since the surgery was performed right into the visible cyst wall.

Case 2

A 41-year-old patient presented with swelling in the eye for a year. He had a history of an episode of acute inflammation followed by swelling, for which he received some treatment. The acute inflammation recovered, but the swelling had remained. The patient was concerned because the swelling was unsightly.

TECHNIQUE

Anesthesia

Administer subconjunctival lignocaine 2%.

Surgical Technique

1. In our case, the swelling was located toward the medical canthus. Because of the severe fibrotic reaction, we could not correctly locate the center of the cyst, so we made an incision parallel to the limbus and about 10 mm away from it failed to reveal the cyst. Clearly we had missed the cyst. We decided to cut the conjunctiva and look underneath.

2. A large Fugo blade incision was made close to the limbus and the conjunctival edges were separated. We could now frankly palpate the cyst. An incision was made over it perpendicular to the limbus. The incision was right on the correct spot, because the cyst began to extrude, but it was firmly attached to the sclera and had to be removed in pieces.

3. No adjacent tissue was excised and the conjunctiva was closed with sutures (Fig. 16.2).

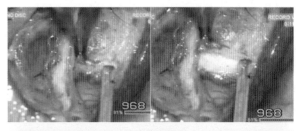
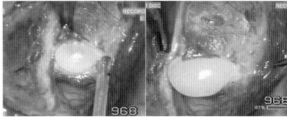

Figure 16.2. The first vertical incision failed to expose the cyst. A large conjunctival incision was then made that located the cyst. The cyst was opened with a horizontal incision.

Postoperative Management

Our patient had an uneventful recovery.

Summary

The Fugo blade incises without causing bleeding. Its ablative cutting action is precise and allows the cystic balloon to extrude without rupturing. If further maneuvers to remove the cyst lead to rupture, the cyst can be easily removed in pieces.

Suggested Reading

Bansal RK, Gupta A, Grewal SP, et al. Spontaneous extrusion of cysticercosis: report of three cases. *Indian J Ophthalmol.* 1992;40:59–60.

Kapoor S, Kapoor MS. Ocular cysticercosis. *J Pediatr Ophthalmol Strabismus.* 1978;15:170–173.

Mohan K, Saroha V, Sharma A, et al. Extraocular muscle cysticercosis: clinical presentations and outcome of treatment. *J Pediatr Ophthalmol Strabismus.* 2005;42:28–33.

Murthy GR, Rao AV. Sub-conjunctival cysticercosis. *Indian J Ophthalmol.* 1980;28:77–78.

Sundaram PM, Jayakumar N, Noronha V. Extraocular muscle cysticercosis—a clinical challenge to the ophthalmologists. *Orbit.* 2004;23:255–262.

Part D
The Lens

Thick Pupillary Membranes

RAVIJIT SINGH

Surgical management of thick iridocapsular membranes is difficult. At times, these membranes may be so tough that it becomes difficult if not impossible to cut them with a capsulotomy needle, a small scissors, or a vitrectomy cutter. Although originally designed as a capsulotomy device, the Fugo blade is an invaluable cutting device for the management of thick iridocapsular membranes. In cases of ocular trauma, persistent hyaloid vasculature, or membranes thickened as a result of postoperative complications, the use of the Fugo blade is amply justified.

We have successfully used the Fugo blade to perform membranectomy inside the anterior chamber.

TECHNIQUE

Anesthesia

Inject topical drops or lidocaine under the conjunctiva.

Surgical Technique

1. Make a 2.8-mm keratome incision at the limbus and a paracentesis incision at 90 degrees from this incision.

2. Deepen the anterior chamber with hydroxypropylmethylcellulose (HPMC). Introduced the plasma knife tip at the 2.8-mm incision.

3. Use the paracentesis incision to continuously inject methyl cellulose into the anterior chamber while the knife is cutting. This helps keep the anterior chamber deep and aids in pushing the cavitation bubbles away from the working field. To this end, a 26-gauge cannula connected via a silicone tube to an HPMC syringe is used, operated by an assistant on instruction from the surgeon. This method offers more control than having the surgeon alone trying to inject the HPMC. In addition, the HPMC cannula helps to stabilize the globe while the Fugo blade is in action.

4. Once the HPMC irrigating cannula is in place and the tip of the plasma knife is positioned inside the anterior chamber, calculate the size of the opening. Usually one pass is enough to cut the membrane through its entire thickness. Cut any bridges of uncut tissue with a second pass.

5. Stain the anterior capsule or the membrane with trypan blue to provide extra visibility. Pupil-dilating hooks may be needed in certain cases to achieve suitable exposure of the surgical field.

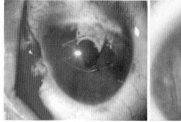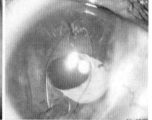

Figure 17.2. The same patient as in Figure 17.1 at the end of surgery **(left)** and 10 months later **(right)**.

CASE STUDIES

Case 1: Posttraumatic Thick Pupillary Membrane

A 22-year-old man suffered an injury in a road accident 6 months prior. The left eye was lost and the right eye suffered severe injuries. The cornea had been repaired. The ruptured cataract had absorbed, leaving behind a thick membrane in the pupil formed by the fusion of the anterior and posterior capsules and imprisoned lens material. We planned to clear the visual axis with the plasma knife and implant an iris claw lens, if possible.

After making the usual entry points the plasma knife tip was introduced into the anterior chamber through a 2.8-mm keratome incision while the HPMC cannula was introduced from the left paracentesis to deliver continuous methylcellulose irrigation (Fig. 17.1).

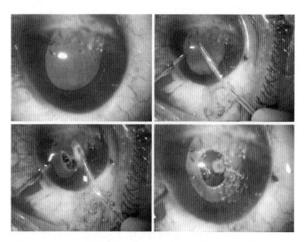

Figure 17.1. Thick posttraumatic pupillary membrane (Case 1) is cut with the Fugo blade.

The Fugo blade was activated and a round circle was traced and cut in the optical axis of the dense membrane, followed by a small anterior vitrectomy.

An iris claw lens was implanted (Fig. 17.2) and fixed to the anterior surface of the iris.

Case 2: Capsulotomy for Congenital Cataract

A 9-year-old patient had had surgery for congenital cataract and posterior chamber lens 4 years before. We used the Fugo blade to perform capsulotomy.

The pupil was pulled in one direction and then dilated with iris hooks. The intra-ocular lens was found to be encapsulated with thick membrane on both sides. Membranectomy of the dense membranes on both sides was performed with great ease, using the Fugo blade at medium settings (Figs. 17.3 and 17.4).

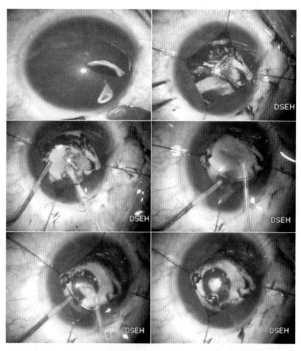

Figure 17.3. Postcataract surgery as a complicated case (Case 2). The iris is retracted and the Fugo blade is taken under the optic of the posterior chamber lens and a round membranectomy is done.

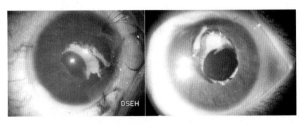

Figure 17.4. The same patient as in Figure 17.3, showing the appearance at the end of surgery (left) and 4 months later (right).

Case 3: Pupilloplasty

We performed a pupilloplasty on a 12-year-old patient who had a traumatic cataract with a posterior chamber lens.

As a result of surgery to correct a congenital cataract 4 years earlier, the patient showed pupil capture, a dense membrane, and pupil shrinkage and deformation. There was only one loop of the lens; the other was missing. We first attempted to remove the membrane using a vitrector, but were not successful. We also tried using a capsulotomy needle, but this too failed, and the tissue began to bleed. Finally, the intimidating vascularized iridocapsular membrane in the pupillary area was managed with the Fugo blade. A perfect pupilloplasty was performed, followed by a small anterior vitrectomy. The appearance and recovery were good (Fig. 17.5).

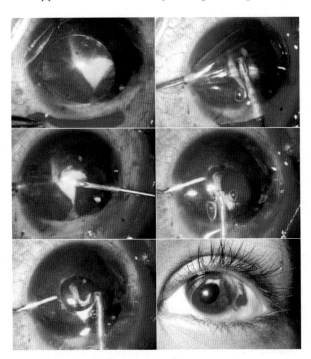

Figure 17.5. Pupil capture and dense membrane formation. First a vitrector was tried and then capsulotomy was attempted with a needle, but both failed. Finally, the Fugo blade was used to do a clean membranectomy and pupilloplasty. The final photo was taken 20 days after surgery.

Case 4: Thick Congenital Vascularized Membrane

One of the toughest challenges in cataract surgery is the management of vascular membranes. These vascular membranes are not only tough to cut but also notorious for bleeding.

Figure 17.6 is the B-scan ultrasound of a 7-month-old patient with a unilateral cataract. The child did not allow detailed examination in the outpatient department but the B-scan revealed the presence of a thick oblique band extending from the back of the lens to the area of the disc. Undoubtedly this was a case of persistent hyaloid vasculature leading to opacification of the lenticular tissue. Based on our previous experience, we expected to encounter some vascularization.

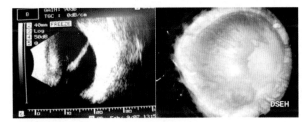

Figure 17.6. A profusely vascularized congenital cataract B-scan showed a thick oblique band from the lens to the retina.

In surgery, we encountered a dense white cataract that was heavily vascularized (Fig. 17.7). The anterior capsule of the cataract was stained with trypan blue and a combination of a capsulotome and a capsularexsis (Utrata) forceps was used to do an irregular capsulotomy. Part fluffy and part stony-type cortex was removed with an irrigation/aspiration (I/A) cannula and a forceps.

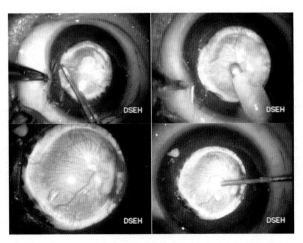

Figure 17.7. Anterior capsulotomy is done, followed by irrigation with aspiration. The thick vascularized posterior capsule is exposed.

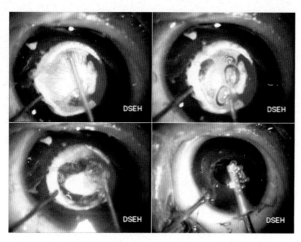

Figure 17.8. The capsulotomy of the vascularized membrane was done with the Fugo blade, followed by clearance with a vitrector.

Once the cortex was removed, the real picture emerged. The posterior capsule was very thick and profusely vascularized, and all the blood vessels appeared to emerge from a single point, presumably at the point of attachment of the persistent hyaloid vessels (Fig. 17.8).

When the Fugo blade was activated, the cutting was instantaneous; however, at places the membrane was so thick than the full length of the cutting tip was unable to penetrate it, so a second pass was needed to incise it all the way. We were surprised to note that despite the number of blood vessels cut, there was minimal bleeding from the tissues. The portion of the membrane that was the node of all the blood vessels bled a bit more than the rest. The cord of persistent hyaloid vasculature could be clearly visualized attached to the back of the posterior capsule.

Finally, the last part of the membrane was cleared away with a vitreous cutter.

Summary

The Fugo blade has proven to be a capable cutting instrument. Its impeccable cutting ability along with its hemostatic properties makes it an excellent choice for the treatment of thick pupillary membranes.

Suggested Reading

Fugo RJ. Fugo blade to enlarge phimotic capsulorrhexis. *J Cataract Refract Surg.* 2006;32:1900.

Samalonis LB. Improving capsulotomies. *Eyeworld.* 2001; 6:42–44.

Singh SK. Fugo blade capsulotomy: a new tech cutting technology. *Trop Ophthalmol.* 2001;1:14–16.

Cataracts and Capsulorrhexis RICHARD J. FUGO

Capsulorrhexis has been the most favored form of capsulotomy over the past two decades.[1] Capsulorrhexis produces the strongest capsulotomy rim of any capsulotomy to date because it produces a continuous tear within normal tissue planes. But capsulorrhexis is not without its limitations.

First, the surgeon attempts to tear a round opening in a convex surface. The force vector on the surface of a convex structure is toward the peripheral equator of the lens; the surgeon counters this by pulling the tear toward the center of the lens. If the tear slips into the periphery, then we have a surgical crisis. Two of the issues that cause problems with capsulorrhexis include poor visibility and raised intracapsular pressure. The total force or pressure that the nucleus and cortex place on the internal surface of the lens capsule is directly related to the surface area of the anterior capsule. Because the area of the lens capsule is πr^2, the diameter of the capsulotomy has a high impact on the total force placed against the rim of the lens capsulotomy. Recall that the total force placed on the internal surface of the anterior capsule is related to the square of the radius of the capsulotomy. For this reason, 7-mm capsulotomy results in an immense decrease in the total force on the internal surface of the anterior capsule rim as compared with 5-mm capsulotomy. Therefore, the risk of a tear of the anterior capsule rim in 7-mm capsulotomy is much lower than that in 5-mm capsulotomy. A 7-mm Fugo blade capsulotomy is easy and safe, whereas 7-mm capsulorrhexis carries a high risk of a tear into the periphery. Poor visibility is a minimal risk with a Fugo blade capsulotomy because it is quite easy to perform Fugo blade capsulotomy under the iris out of direct visualization of the surgeon.[2] This also allows maximum control over corneal pathology, such as Saltzman nodular degeneration. Complicated surgeries such as floppy iris syndrome are much more controlled and made safer using Fugo plasma ablation rather than capsulorrhexis, because Fugo blade capsulotomy can be created under the uncooperative iris out of view of the surgeon.[3,4] Furthermore, standard capsulorrhexis creates postoperative complications such as capsule retention syndrome and capsular phimosis.[5] These pathologies are all but eliminated with a large Fugo blade capsulotomy. Fugo blade capsulotomy offers significant advantages over standard capsulorrhexis. Unlike standard diathermy, a Fugo blade capsulotomy provides rim strength that is close to that of standard capsulorrhexis.[6,7] Ophthalmologists finally have an alternative to performing capsulorrhexis.

References

1. Gimbel HV, Neuhann T. Continuous curvilinear capsulorrhexis. *J Cataract Refract Surg.* 1991;17:110–111.
2. Fugo RJ, DelCampo DM. The Fugo blade™: the next step after capsulorrhexis. *Ann Ophthalmol.* 2001;33:12–20.
3. Ronge L. How to use the Fugo blade. *EyeNet.* 2003; 7:23–24.
4. Young M. Fugo blade finds its niche in difficult cases. *Eyeworld.* 2003;8:70.
5. Sabbagh LB. Rhexis can hold IOL when posterior capsule breaks. *Ocular Surgery News.* 1992;3:1–10.
6. Wilson ME, Trivedi RH. Technological advances make pediatric cataract surgery safer and faster. *Tech Ophthalmol.* 2003;1:53–61.
7. Wilson ME. Anterior lens capsule management in pediatric cataract surgery. *Trans Am Ophthalmol Soc.* 2004;102:391–422.

19 Capsulotomy in Difficult Cataracts KIRANJIT SINGH

Soon after I entered the field of phaco-emulsification, I began hearing about the problems surgeons had managing a difficult type of cataract called "posterior polar cataract," which consisted of typical concentric rings around the central lenticular opacity (onion ring). Review of the literature revealed that standard treatment was to perform a regular 5.5-mm circular central capsulorrhexis and not to perform hydrodissection. In the subsequent months I treated many such cases with equal success (avoiding posterior capsule rupture) and failure (posterior capsule opening with or without the lens dropping into the vitreous). I wondered what was lacking in my technique and concluded that scarcity of working area led to failures. So I increased the size of the capsulotomy in one direction, the direction of sculpting. What resulted was a complete absence of posterior capsule ruptures and nucleus drops, not only in posterior polar cataracts but also in cases with preexisting ruptures. More importantly, surgical time was cut in half. I extended my experience with long oval capsulotomy to hard cataracts and found it to be equally effective.

Two difficult situations for a phaco-emulsification surgeon are posterior polar cataracts and white cataracts. A posterior polar cataract is a dense, white, rounded opacity situated on the central posterior capsule that typically consists of concentric rings around the central opacity. It has an inherent tendency to present with posterior capsule rupture either during surgery or even before it as a preexisting posterior capsular rent. Osher and colleagues (1990) reported a 26% (8 of 31 eyes) incidence of posterior capsule rupture during surgery in eyes with a posterior polar cataract.[1]

To prevent posterior capsular rupture, various measures have been suggested in the literature, including slow-motion phaco-emulsification with low aspiration flow rate, a low level of vacuum and infusion pressure; viscodissection to immobilize epinucleus and cortex; and inside-out delineation.

Large Oval Capsulotomy

I use a large oval capsulotomy or capsulorrhexis from the 12 o'clock periphery to the 6 o'clock periphery to treat all cases of posterior polar cataract. This technique has all but eliminated posterior capsule rupture. Several advantages to this type of capsulotomy are:

- It guards against accidental increase of in-the-bag pressure during water-powered procedures.
- It increases the working area so that sculpting can be done in the entire length of the nucleus, which aids easy division.
- It facilitates easy removal of lens fragments with the bimanual help of the phaco probe and the chopper without any rotatory movement (which needs to be avoided).
- Shorter sides of the rhexis function like a tamponade to the forward-bulging vitreous mushroom.
- The maneuverability while performing a posterior circular central capsulorrhexis is improved because of the greater working area.
- Large oval capsulotomy gives a stronger grip to optic capture of the 6-mm intra-ocular lens to be

implanted in the sulcus in case in-the-bag implantation appears risky.

- Plenty of space between the optic edge and capsulotomy edge means a vitrectomy probe can be introduced without tilting the intra-ocular lens.

The large oval capsulotomy is useful when the diagnosis of a pre-existing posterior capsule rupture is suspected or established. To illustrate the utility of large oval capsulotomy, I have chosen an even more complicated case than a posterior polar cataract. In this case, pre-existing posterior capsular rupture was suspected.

TECHNIQUE

Anesthesia

The patient was given peribulbar anesthesia with pressure on the eyeball to make the globe soft.

Surgical Technique

1. Make two ports, one side port at the 1 o'clock position and a second phaco port at 11 o'clock.
2. Stain the anterior capsule with trypan blue for better visibility, then fill the anterior chamber with visco-elastic material.
3. Use a Fugo blade to make a large oval capsulotomy in a vertical direction (Fig. 19.1).
4. Start phaco-emulsification of the nucleus. At the end of it, you will see a rent in the posterior

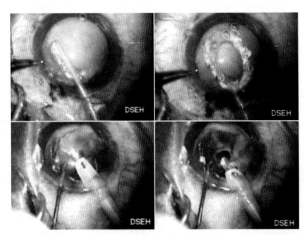

Figure 19.1. A long vertically oval capsulotomy is made with the Fugo blade. The nucleus is removed. When the torn posterior capsule becomes visible through the cortex, phaco-emulsification is stopped.

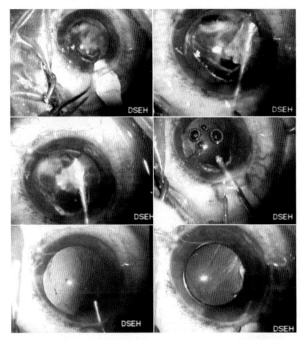

Figure 19.2. The main incision is enlarged and the area is aspirated manually. When the vitreous appears, a vitrector is used. The posterior chamber intra-ocular lens is implanted in the bag. The long posterior capsular rent is visible under the intra-ocular lens.

capsule, through a gap in the cortex. Withdraw the phaco-emulsification probe.

5. Extend the phacoemulsification incision (Fig. 19.2).
6. Use dry aspiration in the capsular bag to clear the cortex.
7. Perform a small anterior vitrectomy.
8. Implant a posterior chamber intra-ocular lens inside the capsular bag. In our case, the edge of the posterior capsular tear and the anterior capsulotomy were visible.

During our procedure there was no extension of the posterior capsular tear. The long oval Fugo blade capsulotomy prevents pressure build-up inside the capsular bag. It also allows the phaco-emulsification process to be done along a greater length of the nucleus than would be allowed if the capsulotomy was a standard circular 5.5 mm.

Large Round Capsulotomy in a White Cataract

Fugo blade capsulotomy makes it simple to make a large capsulotomy. No capsulotomy is extended toward the periphery, which could threaten the posterior capsule (Fig.19.3).

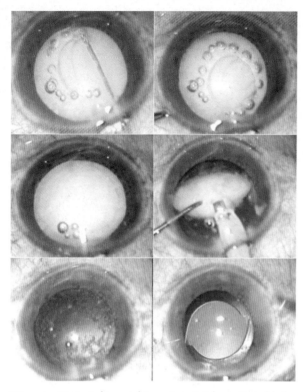

Figure 19.3. A dense white cataract. A large Fugo blade capsulotomy makes it easy to bring out and perform phaco-emulsification on the hard lens. The lens matter is aspirated. A posterior chamber intra-ocular lens has been implanted, without covering the anterior capsule.

It is commonly taught that Elschnig pearls develop as a result of anterior epithelial cell migration from under the anterior capsule onto the posterior capsule. If this is true, then why do we preserve the anterior capsule? If preservation of the anterior capsule has something to do with holding the optic tight and pushing it back against the posterior capsule to prevent after-cataract formation, why does the credit for a postoperative clean posterior capsule go to certain type of lens design? I think that an intra-ocular lens with a square edge prevents posterior capsular opacification even in the absence of a leatherlike anterior capsule.

Summary

Large oval capsulotomy using the Fugo blade has several advantages. With a large capsulotomy, the phobia about posterior polar and hard cataracts is gone.

Risk to the integrity of the superior or the inferior margin of capsulotomy during phaco-emulsification is reduced to nothing. With an increased working area and increased gutter length, the bimanual force applied in opposite directions to break the segments is reduced, which helps safeguard weak zonules. Despite the use of high phaco power to emulsify stonelike cataracts, the incidence and severity of striate keratitis have been reduced.

Reference

1. Osher RH, Yu BC, Koch DD. Posterior polar cataracts: a predisposition to intraoperative posterior capsular rupture. *J. Cataract Refract Surg.* 1990;16:157–162.

Suggested Readings

Allen D, Wood C. Minimizing risk to the capsule during surgery for posterior polar cataract. *J Cataract Refract Surg.* 2002;28:742–744.

Anis AY. Understanding hydrodelineation: the term and the procedure. *Doc Ophthalmol.* 1994;87:123–137.

Consultation section: cataract surgical problem. *J Cataract Refract Surg.* 1997;23:819–824.

Emery JM, Little JH. *Phacoemulsification and aspiration of cataracts, surgical technique, complications and results.* St. Louis, Mo: Mosby, 1979:45–49.

Fine IH. Cortico-cleaving hydrodissection. *J Cataract Refract Surg.* 1992;18:508–512.

Fine IH, Packer M, Hoffman RS. Management of posterior polar cataract. *J Cataract Refract Surg.* 2003;29:16–19.

Gimbel HV, DeBroff BM. Posterior capsulorrhexis with optic capture: maintaining a clear visual axis after pediatric cataract surgery. *J Cataract Refract Surg.* 1994;20:658–664.

Osher RH. Slow motion phacoemulsification approach. *J Cataract Refract Surg.* 1993;19:667.

Osher RH, Cionni R, Burk S. Intraoperative complications of phacoemulsification surgery. In: Steinert RH, ed. *Cataract surgery: technique. complications. and management.* 2nd ed. Philadelphia, Pa: Saunders, 2004:469–486

Vasavada AR, Desai JP. Stop, chop, chop, and stuff. *J Cataract Refract Surg.* 1996;22:526–529.

Vasavada AR, Irivedi R. Role of optic capture in congenital cataract and IOL surgery in children. *J Cataract Refract Surg.* 2000;26:824–831.

Vasavada AR, Raj SM. Inside-out delineation. *J Cataract Refract Surg.* 2004;30:1167–1169.

Vasavada AR, Singh R. Phacoemulsification with posterior polar cataract. *J Cataract Refract Surg.* 1999;25:238–245.

Vasavada AR, Singh R. Step-by-step chop in situ and separation of very dense cataracts. *J Cataract Refract Surg.* 1998;24:156–159.

8-mm Capsulotomy RICHARD J. FUGO

The phrase "8-mm capsulotomy" is only a general description. The description means that we create a capsulotomy much larger than a standard 5.5-mm capsulotomy (Fig. 20.1). The precise size of the large capsulotomy varies according to the size of the eye. In sum, I make a capsulotomy 2 mm from the limbus. Many would say that this will damage zonules, but close analysis shows that this is not the case.[1]

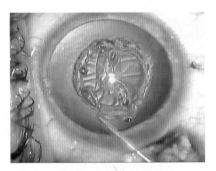

Figure 20.1. A standard 5.5-mm Fugo blade capsulotomy is created in about 6 seconds.

Over the course of 10 years, I have performed several thousand of these large capsulotomies and yet have not had a single subluxation of an intraocular lens. From a pathophysiologic point of view, we should study patients with aniridia. In these patients, the tips of the ciliary processes extend inward toward the center of the eye such that the innermost tip of the ciliary processes reach the limbus, except on the temporal aspect of the eye, where they extend about 0.75 to 1 mm past the limbus. Because I am surgeon who performs temporal incision cataract surgery, I can easily achieve a capsulotomy 2 mm from the limbus everywhere except at the tem-poral aspect of the eye, where I can achieve a capsulotomy about 3 mm in from the limbus (Fig. 20.2). This procedure works out perfectly because the ciliary processes extend further inward at the temporal aspect of the eye.

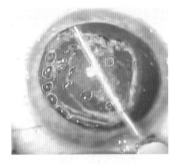

Figure 20.2. It is simple to enlarge a capsulotomy with the Fugo blade. An 8-mm capsulotomy is being created around the 5.5-mm capsulotomy shown in Figure 20.1 with the Fugo blade tip under the iris out of view of the surgeon.

An 8-mm mechanical capsulorrhexis is very difficult to achieve without risk into the periphery. Yet, the 8-mm capsulotomy offers distinct advantages over the 5.5-mm capsulotomy.[2] The large capsulotomy results in minimal force on the anterior capsule leaflet, thus reducing the risk of tearing the anterior capsule rim. A large capsulotomy all but eliminates anterior capsule contraction syndrome and capsule retention syndrome. I have observed that the small anterior capsule rim begins binding to the posterior capsule in 4 to 8 weeks postoperatively, thereby locking the haptics in place and preventing anterior capsule phimosis.

Because the lens is a convex structure, ablating the capsulotomy 2 mm from the limbus based on the surgeon's view through the operating microscope actually produces a much wider rim than is seen from the surgeon's view. This is because the surgeon is seeing a flat view of a structure that actually exists on an angle.

TECHNIQUE

The 8-mm capsulotomy allows a surgeon to quickly remove the lens nucleus from the lens bag.[3] An 8-mm capsulotomy can easily be performed under the iris out of view of the surgeon as well as with a cloudy cornea (see Chapter 21: Small Pupil Cataract Surgery).

Surgical Technique

1. Once you have completed an 8-mm capsulotomy, perform hydrodissection.
2. Then use the phaco tip to impale the nucleus, rock it gently, and pluck it out of the lens bag.
3. At this point, inject visco-elastic material behind the nucleus to push the posterior capsule back and to hold the nucleus in the pupil, where it can be mechanically cracked and phaco-emulsification performed (Fig. 20.3).

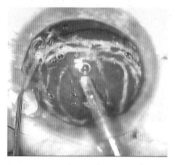

Figure 20.3. With the nucleus impaled with the phaco tip, it is lifted out of the lens bag while a viscoelastic cannula on the left places a cushion of viscoelastic material behind the nucleus.

By removing the nucleus from the lens bag, the surgeon proceeds with surgery while eliminating stress on lens zonules and minimizing risk to the posterior capsule. This technique is extremely important in cases with weak zonules such as pseudo-exfoliation.[4]

It should be emphasized that a Fugo blade capsulotomy can be performed in one continuous movement or can be created by joining multiple arcuate capsulotomy maneuvers (Fig. 20.4). This allows the surgeon to impale the nucleus with the phaco tip and pluck the nucleus out of the lens bag, then mechanically crack the nucleus in the iris plane (Figs. 20.5 and 20.6).

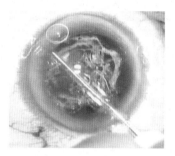

Figure 20.4. Multiple accurate capsulotomies are utilized to create an 8-mm capsulotomy in a different patient. Here the Fugo blade is under the iris in the process of creating accurate capsulotomies that are joined to create a final 8-mm capsulotomy.

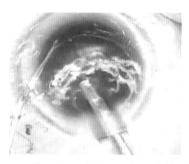

Figure 20.5. The phaco tip is used to pluck the nucleus out of the lens bag of the patient seen in Figure 20.4 while viscoelastic material is being injected behind the nucleus with the side-port cannula to push the posterior capsule back and hold the nucleus in the iris plane.

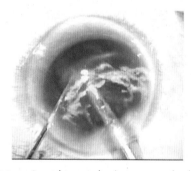

Figure 20.6. A nucleus probe is seen on the left being pushed through the body of the nucleus until it hits the phaco tip, thereby mechanically cracking the nucleus in the iris plane.

Summary

The 8-mm capsulotomy has realistic advantages for the surgeon. However, achieving a repeatable, safe 8-mm capsulorrhexis is difficult because a capsule tear that approaches the equator of the lens carries a high risk of escaping outward to the equator based on force vectors that aim the capsule tear toward the lens equator. On the other hand, plasma ablation of the anterior capsule with the Fugo blade allows a safe, repeatable 8-mm capsulotomy that may be created in one pass or in multiple passes.[5] A microscopic view of a Fugo blade ablation path shows "rounded" ends that lack an acute nidus, and are therefore not prone to spontaneous tearing. Capsulorrhexis, on the other hand, has acute angles at the end of each tear in the capsule, which provides the perfect nidus for continued spontaneous tearing.[6]

Fugo blade plasma ablation is a paradigm shift in cataract surgery. Powered by C-cell rechargeable batteries, its low energy output is the foundation for its unparalleled safety profile even with weakened corneas or weakened zonules. Most importantly, the Fugo plasma blade allows the surgeon to perform surgeries that were previously almost impossible to perform without this novel technology.[7]

References

1. Kent C. Minimizing zonular stress with the plasma blade. *Ophthalmol Manage*. 2004;8:157.
2. Fugo RJ. Mature cataracts: how to breeze through them. *Ocular Surg News*. 2006;24:8–9.
3. Fugo R. Cushioned PhacoXcap technique addresses difficulties with small pupils, hard cataracts. *Ocular Surg News*. 2005;23:16–17.
4. Kent C. PhacoXcap: a new procedure makes it possible to phaco both nucleus & cortex outside the capsular bag. *Ophthalmol Manage*. 2002;6:80.
5. Charters L. Cataract surgeons gain better control with capsulotomy blade. *Ophthalmol Times*. 2003;28:16.
6. Fugo RJ, DelCampo DM. The Fugo blade™: the next step after capsulorrhexis. *Ann Ophthalmol*. 2001;33:12–20.
7. Video journal of cataract & refractive surgery. *New Dev New Devices Fugo Blade*. 2002;18(1).

21 Small-Pupil Cataract Surgery RICHARD J. FUGO

A hallmark of modern cataract surgery is excellent visualization with a modern coaxial operating microscope. As with any biologic phenomenon, dilation of the pupil can be quantitated by placing it on a bell-shaped curve. My colleagues and I have noted that some patients' eyes maximally dilate with one set of dilating eye drops whereas others barely dilate with a large series of dilating eye drops. Patients on alpha-antagonists such as tamsulosin, alfuzosin, terazosin, and doxazosin manifest poor dilation with an "irrational" acting iris during cataract surgery, such as a billowing iris. This phenomenon is known as "floppy iris syndrome"[1] (Fig. 21.1). The surgeon can stretch the iris when performing a Fugo blade capsulotomy because the nucleus is removed from the lens bag and lodged in the pupil. Herein, the nucleus acts to stabilize the iris while the phaco tip is meticulously disassembling the nucleus (Figs. 21.2 and 21.3) Corneal opacity such as seen in Salzmann nodular degeneration is also a challenge for modern cataract surgery because it poses an obstruction to visualization.

Many types of iris retraction devices can mechanically dilate the iris.[2–5] All of these devices have issues

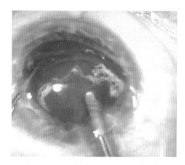

Figure 21.2. The nucleus in Figure 21.1 is impaled with the phaco tip, which is used to pluck it out of the lens bag while visco-elastic material is injected behind the nucleus with a side port cannula.

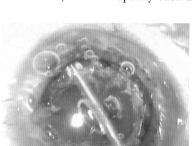

Figure 21.1. A pupil with floppy iris syndrome has been stretched and an 8-mm capsulotomy is being created under the iris out of the surgeon's view.

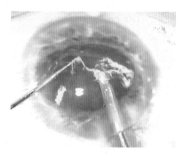

Figure 21.3. A pool of visco-elastic material acts to hold up the nucleus in the pupil, thereby acting to stabilize this iris as the nucleus is meticulously disassembled in the iris plane.

such as cost, lengthening the time of surgery, corneal trauma, and iris trauma. Iris retraction with micromanipulator probes is often helpful, but it provides limited dilation.[6,7] A large superior sector iridectomy is often helpful, but it can cause an undesirable cosmetic outcome.[8] Small incisions scattered along the pupil margin require expensive micro-scissors and produce only a moderate increase in pupil dilation. This approach can cause bleeding and significantly increase surgical time.

The Fugo blade offers a new dimension in the management of small-pupil cataract surgery.[9] The Fugo blade allows the surgeon to ablate anterior capsule under the iris out of view of the surgeon.[10] Because I prefer large capsulotomies, I perform about 40% of my capsulotomies under the iris without any visualization of the capsulotomy. The learning curve for this maneuver is quite low, while the outcome is truly invaluable.[11]

Surgical Technique

1. Infuse visco-elastic between the iris and capsule to lift the iris off the anterior capsule 360 degrees.

2. Introduce the Fugo blade tip into the anterior chamber and begin ablating the capsule within the pupil, then slowly continue the ablation outward under the iris. You will see the iris surface mildly tent up as the Fugo blade tip passes under a given point of the iris (Fig. 21.4).

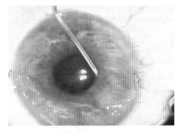

Figure 21.4. A Fugo blade is seen under a constricted iris while an 8-mm capsulotomy is ablated out of the surgeon's view.

3. Do *not* move the Fugo blade under the iris if the tip is not activated because this risks a mechanical tear in the capsule.

4. Perform capsule ablation in one continuous maneuver or in several connected arcuate maneuvers that begin and end within the pupil, thereby beginning with visualization and ending with visualization.

5. A major risk of Fugo plasma capsulotomy is to leave a skip lesion in the capsule, resulting in the capsulotomy not being a complete 360-degree

ablation but rather a peninsula-shaped skip area attached to the central capsule island created with the Fugo blade. To eliminate skip lesions, I perform three or four 360-degree capsulotomies at the same general location on the capsule. I perform each in a slow and deliberate manner, requiring about 30 seconds each. If a skip lesion in the capsule is left when phaco begins, removal of the central capsule island may cause the island to tear out peripherally toward the equator.

6. Since I routinely use a large capsulotomy, I can impale the nucleus with the phaco tip and rock it out of the lens bag (Fig. 21.5). I normally ablate the capsule at a distance of 2 mm from the limbus. This leaves a small but healthy capsule rim with no significant damage to the zonules. Be sure to hydrodissect prior to impaling the nucleus with the phaco tip.

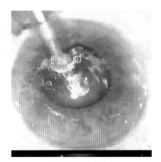

Figure 21.5. After an 8-mm capsulotomy formation, the phaco tip is used to impale the nucleus to lift it out of the lens bag as well as having the nucleus stretch the pupil open.

7. Once the nucleus is out of the lens bag and still on the phaco tip, a visco-elastic cannula can be inserted through a cornea side stab incision and visco-elastic material can be injected behind the nucleus to push the posterior capsule backward and hold the nucleus in the pupil after it is released from the phaco tip (Fig. 21.6).

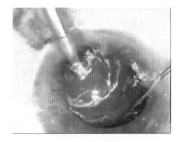

Figure 21.6. The impaled nucleus is used to pull the pupil open while visco-elastic material is injected behind it to hold the nucleus up in the pupil.

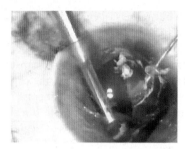

Figure 21.7. Held in the pupil on a cushion of visco-elastic material, the nucleus is mechanically cracked in the iris plane with the phaco tip and the nucleus manipulator.

8. The nucleus acts to hold the pupil open as you mechanically crack it, then you perform phaco-emulsification on the cracked piece of nucleus in the iris plane (Fig. 21.7).

Summary

This Fugo blade technique dramatically simplifies cataract surgery in small-pupil cases. Once a surgeon learns this procedure, he or she will be able to take control of those difficult small-pupil cataract cases (Figs. 21.8 and 21.9).

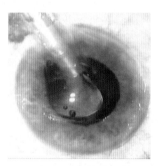

Figure 21.8. Once the nucleus and cortex are removed, the intra-ocular lens is unfolded into the lens bag.

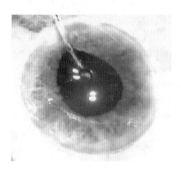

Figure 21.9. The intra-ocular lens (IOL) is being moved back and forth with the IOL manipulator to check for haptic spring and IOL centration. In this case, the observed results are excellent.

References

1. Chang DF, Campbell JR. The intraoperative floppy iris syndrome associated with tamsulosin. *Cataract Refract Surg Today.* 2005;31:664–673.
2. De Juan E, Hickingbotham D. Flexible iris retractor. *Am J Ophthalmol.* 1991;111:776–777.
3. Fine IH. Phacoemulsification in the presence of a small pupil. In: Steinert RF, ed. *Cataract surgery: technique, complications and management.* Philadelphia, Pa: Saunders, 1995:199–208.
4. Mackool RJ. Small pupil enlargement during cataract extraction: a new method. *J Cataract Refract Surg.* 1992;18:523–526.
5. Nichamin LD. Enlarging the pupil for cataract extraction using flexible nylon iris retractors. *J Cataract Refract Surg.* 1993;19:793–796.
6. Miller KM, Kenner GT. Stretch pupilloplasty for small pupil phacoemulsification. *Am J Ophthalmol.* 1994;3:107–108.
7. Dinsmore SC. Modified stretch technique for small pupil phacoemulsification with topical anesthesia. *J Cataract Surg.* 1996;22:27–30.
8. Lu LW, Fine IH. *Phacoemulsification in difficult and challenging cases.* New York: Thieme, 1999.
9. Fugo RJ, DelCampo DM. The Fugo blade™: the next step after capsulorrhexis. *Ann Ophthalmol.* 2001;33:12–20.
10. Fugo RJ, Singh D, Fine IH. Automated Fugo blade capsulotomy: a new technique and a new instrument. *Eyeworld.* 2002;7:49–54.
11. Fugo RJ. Strategy for capsulotomy. *Cataract Refract Surg Today.* 2007;7:15.

Pediatric Capsulotomy DALJIT SINGH

22

My colleagues and I started performing pediatric lens implantations in 1981; our first case was one of a case of traumatic cataract. Through 2009, over 11,000 pediatric cataracts have been treated. The strategy of cataract surgery then and now has been the same: to remove as much of the anterior capsule as possible, making it easier to remove the cataract and reduce the incidence and severity of secondary cataract formation. Earlier it was the can opener capsulotomy that met our needs. Now we use the Fugo blade. Our lens of choice has been an iris claw lens since we started. Now the intra-ocular lens is mostly in the bag lens when the capsule is intact and in iris claw lens when the capsule is not intact.

Use of the Fugo blade for pediatric capsulotomy is described and some case examples are explained.

Surgical Technique

1. Make two incisions: A small one through which to pass the visco-elastic cannula, and a large one through which to introduce the intra-ocular lens (Fig. 22.1).

2. Keep the anterior chamber deep throughout the procedure, so that the endothelium is not touched.

3. Start the capsulotomy at any point on the capsule, with the Fugo blade's energy setting at the lowest. The movement of the capsulotomy draws a line on the capsule, which is removed from the incision line instantly. The length of time needed to complete the incision depends on the surgeon—It may take 1 second or 20 seconds; the result is the same. If any area is been skipped, it can be gotten on a subsequent pass.

4. Remove the cataract, which may be accomplished without difficulty because the aspirating cannula can easily reach the capsular fornices.

Any variety of intra-ocular lens can be implanted with ease.

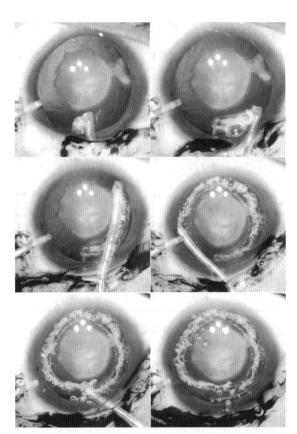

Figure 22.1. Visco-elastic material is injected through the side port, while the Fugo blade tip draws a circular ablation line on the capsule. The ablation process creates a gap between the cut edges.

Whatever the thickness of the capsule, whatever the consistency of the opacification of the cataract, the Fugo blade can open the membrane. Neither red reflex nor staining the capsule with trypan blue is necessary. The cavitation bubbles close to the tip of the Fugo blade provide a perfect visual check on the progress of the capsulotomy. In contrast to manual capsulotomy, with the Fugo blade presents no risk of the capsulotomy running out of control, toward the equator.

CASE STUDIES

Case 1: Capsulotomy in a Pre-existing Posterior Capsule Defect

The cataract in this patient showed a positive Singh sign for a posterior capsular defect (white spots seen in front and around the posterior capsular defect). The Fugo blade capsulotomy did not cause tension or pull that could endanger the extension of posterior capsule defect. The lens was flawlessly extracted manually through the large capsulotomy, and the hole in the posterior capsule remained undisturbed until the end of the surgery (Fig. 22.2).

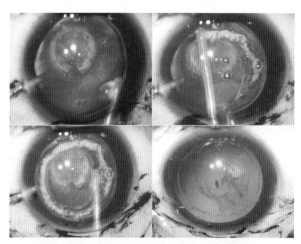

Figure 22.2. In this pre-existing posterior capsular defect (Case 1), a large anterior capsulotomy is performed with a Fugo blade. The posterior capsular hole remains undisturbed until the end of the surgery.

Case 2: Capsulotomy in Marfan Syndrome

Figure 22.3 shows an extreme example of a dislocated lens without zonular support along the inferior border. The pathology did not prevent creation of a suitable capsulotomy through which the lens matter was removed. The capsular bag remained undisturbed until the end of the surgery.

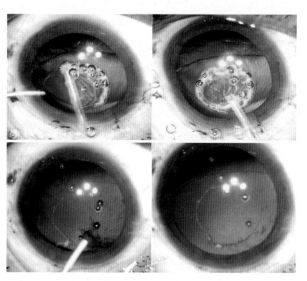

Figure 22.3. In this patient with Marfan syndrome (Case 2), a large capsulotomy was done without resistance, using the Fugo blade. The lens matter was removed without disturbing the capsular bag of the dislocated lens.

Case 3: Posterior Capsulotomy after Secondary Implant

In this case, the thick capsular membrane in the pupillary aperture could have been removed the same way that a primary capsulotomy is done. But using such an approach risked injury to the vitreous beneath the membrane. This capsulotomy was done in a manner that ensured no risk to the vitreous (Fig. 22.4).

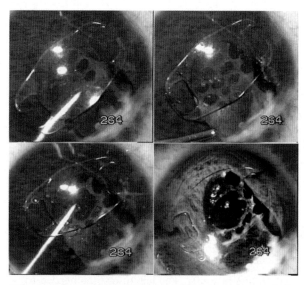

Figure 22.4. In Case 3, the opaque posterior capsule is repeatedly touched with a 300-μm tip to create multiple holes. Uniting some of them in the center creates a fair-sized capsulotomy.

After the artisan lens had been implanted, capsulotomy was begun. A 300-μm Fugo blade tip was used. The undersurface of the tip was stripped of the insulating cover. When activated and touched to the opaque membrane, it created a small hole. Many such holes were created by repeated touch. When joined together, a credible posterior capsulotomy had been produced, with only the slightest damage to the vitreous.

Summary

Performing a capsulotomy in pediatric cases presents numerous challenges, regardless of the etiology—congenital or acquired or the result of trauma or secondary changes. All of these challenges, however, can be met by using the Fugo blade, with minimal trauma and no tissue traction.

Suggested Reading

Singh D, Worst J, Singh R, Singh I R. *Cataract and IOL.* New Delhi. India: Jaypee, 1993.

Singh D, et al. *Pediatric cataract surgery.* Philadelphia, Pa: Lippincott Williams & Wilkins, 2005.

CHAPTER
23

Iridectomy and Iridotomy

DALJIT SINGH

raditionally, a manual iridectomy could be done only after making a suitable incision, inserting a forceps, holding and pulling the iris out of the incision line, and cutting it with scissors. This was followed by irrigation of the anterior chamber and verification of the iris opening. This approach has disadvantages such as bleeding from the iris or from its torn root. The bleeding may be minimal or moderate and rarely massive, and it comes as a shock when it happens in a surgery in which iridectomy was supposed to be a minor component.

Cutting the iris is required in every case of cataract in which any lens other than in-the-bag is to be implanted. It is needed in most cases of traumatic cataract damage following penetrating injury. The iris must also be cut from the adherent leukoma. Pupilloplasty requires extensive cutting of the iris.

In a behind-the-iris phakic lens implantation, iridectomy is needed. This can be done with the yttrium–aluminum–garnet (YAG) laser, but that is often easier said than done. A dark, thick iris responds poorly to laser treatment; it may become inflamed or may close. A reliable iridectomy is one in which the iris tissue is actually removed, before or after phakic lens implantation.

All anterior chamber filtration procedures require a patent iridectomy. It is necessary in pseudophakic pupillary block glaucoma, with or without an iris bombe. If the iris bombe is multiloculated, more than one iridectomy is necessary. In such cases, the usual manual approach will require multiple corneal incisions.

The introduction of the Fugo blade for iridectomy changes the scene completely. Iridectomy can be done in situ by mere "touch-and-ablate," with no bleeding. Multiple iridectomies may be done through tiny incisions or through a single incision. An iridectomy may be done toward the diametrically opposite limbus; for example, if an incision has been made at the 12 o'clock position and the situation demands an iridectomy at 6 o'clock, this can be done by carrying the Fugo blade tip across the pupil to the required point. The only requirement is a deep anterior chamber, which is easily created using a visco-elastic agent. The iridectomy/iridotomy may be the size of a pinpoint or larger. It may be circular or linear. In cases of adherent leukoma, the iris must be separated from the lesion. A properly directed Fugo blade tip can incise the iris effortlessly, such that the iris entangled in adherent leukoma is not pulled or tugged, as would be the case in manual iridotomy. The following two cases illustrate iridectomy in three different situations.

CASE STUDIES

Case 1: Iridectomy in Ab Interno Filtration

The patient shown in Figure 23.1 was undergoing an ab interno filtration procedure. Iridectomy was required.

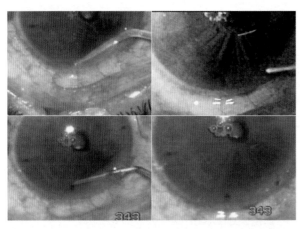

Figure 23.1. Iridectomy before ab interno filtration. The 300-micron Fugo blade tip is activated to ablate the iris. An irrigation cannula verifies the completeness of iridectomy. The cavitation bubbles formed during iridectomy collect under the iris and raise it. Oblique illumination clearly demonstrates this phenomenon.

Surgical Technique

1. Lift the limbal conjunctiva with a visco-elastic material.
2. Make a corneal pocket incision with a diamond knife.
3. Pass a straight 300-μm Fugo blade tip through the pocket incision and touch and slightly press the iris. Set the tip at medium power and energy and activate it momentarily two to three times. This is enough to ablate the iris and create an iris opening.

4. During ablation, cavitation bubbles are produced that get under the iris and raise it. They act as a protective layer against injury to the underlying lens.
5. Directing a light from the side shows the iris elevation clearly. This also ensures that the iris has been breached.
6. Confirm the completeness of iridectomy further by passing an irrigating cannula through the iridectomy. Irrigation also washes out any remaining pigment or iris tissue elements.

Case 2: Iridectomy in Traumatic Cataract

Figure 23.2 shows a young patient with a traumatic cataract in which an anterior chamber lens (iris claw (artisan lens)) had been implanted. Postoperative inflammation led to closure of iridectomy and the pupil. When the patient presented at our clinic, he had severe iris bombe and glaucoma. The anterior chamber was very shallow. This eye was treated as follows.

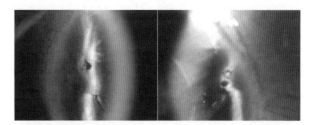

Figure 23.2. A case of pseudophakic pupillary block. A clean-cut iridectomy is made over the temporal claw, and a clear cornea filtration track (close to the iris hole) along with iridectomy is made on the nasal claw.

Surgical Technique

1. Make a pocket incision near the lateral limbus.
2. Introduce a 300-μm Fugo blade tip and perform an iridectomy near the temporal claw of the intraocular lens. The anterior chamber deepens instantly.
3. In our case, the patient's glaucoma also needed management. In a case such as this, perform a transconjunctival anterior chamber filtration on the upper nasal side. Make a clear cornea filtration track with a 300-μm ablating tip. As the ablating tip enters the anterior chamber, it also produces a hole in the iris over the nasal claw.

Postoperative Management

Two months after our surgery, the anterior chamber remained well formed and intra-ocular pressure was 19 mm Hg.

Case 3: Pupilloplasty

Numerous situations arise in which the iris must be ablated to get the desired result. In this case, a 9-year-old child showed an angle-supported lens made out of a posterior chamber lens. There was contraction and occlusion of the pupil and adhesions to the vitreous. This was a situation that is ordinarily not easy to handle. Any manual procedure would cause bleeding from the iris and cause traction to the vitreous. This case was managed as follows (Fig. 23.3).

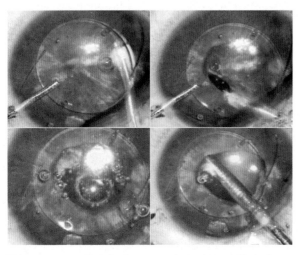

Figure 23.3. An irrigation cannula pushes methylcellulose from the side port, while the capsulotomy tip performs membranectomy-cum-pupilloplasty. The vitrector removes the detritus.

Surgical Technique

1. Make two incisions, one side port for the injection of methylcellulose to keep the anterior chamber deep during the procedure and the other a 2-mm incision to introduce the capsulotomy tip of the Fugo blade.

2. Introduce the capsulotomy tip under the edge of the lens optic, then activate it and move it in a circle twice to perform membranectomy-cum-pupilloplasty.

3. Remove the detritus with a vitrector.

There was no bleeding or traction of the tissues during our procedure.

Summary

In our clinic we have performed countless iridectomies in a variety of clinical situations. I note here three particular precautions for performing iridectomy and iridotomy using the Fugo blade.

- Never work in an anterior chamber that is not constantly deepened with saline or visco-elastic material.
- Never point the Fugo blade tip toward the cornea.
- Never move an inactivated Fugo blade tip inside the iris tissue.

Suggested Reading

Kellan R, Fugo RJ. Device increases safety, efficiency of cataract surgery. *Ophthalmol Times.* 2000;25:7–9.

Roy FH. Course for Fugo blade is enlightening, surgeon says. *Ocular Surg News.* 2001;19:35–38.

Part F
Glaucoma

Glaucoma Surgery DALJIT SINGH

U nlike phaco-emulsification and lens implantation in cataract surgery, no spectacular developments have occurred in glaucoma surgery. Several reasons exist for this.

The basic surgical tools have remained as they were a century ago: forceps, scissors, and knife. Heat cautery has been replaced by bipolar cautery. Lasers are a partial help in a small percentage of cases.

A singular lack of understanding exists regarding the presence and role of conjunctival lymphatics in regulating subconjunctival fluids and their ability to act as flood drains after filtration surgery. Conjunctival lymphatics are rarely mentioned in treatises on glaucoma. Absorption of the draining aqueous is credited either to "filtration" through the conjunctiva, where it mixes with the tear film or to absorption by "vascular or perivascular conjunctival tissue." Exactly what tissue is doing the absorbing is not mentioned. A tissue cannot continue to absorb outflowing aqueous, the aqueous has to drain. Because of the absence of the conjunctival lymphatics on the academic landscape, this fundamental point is missed. Furthermore, new surgical techniques are grossly destructive to conjunctival lymphatics.

Glaucoma surgery has remained focused on drainage from the anterior chamber despite all the postoperative problems that it entails.

The Fugo blade arrived on the scene in 1999. It is held like a pen and cuts like an eximer laser. It makes incisions, gutters, and tracks exactly as required. It ablates blood vessels in its path. At first we used it to perform only the functions required for standard glaucoma surgery. We soon realized, however, that the Fugo blade could perform beyond the limitations of microsurgical instruments and diamond knives.

Use of the Fugo blade revived my interest in addressing drainage from the posterior chamber. Thus came transciliary filtration. Also, the unique nature of the Fugo plasma blade helped in finding newer and perhaps better ways of draining the anterior chamber. Study of conjunctival lymphatics had a direct impact on the development of simpler and less traumatic techniques. Postoperative complications and failures could now be addressed in new and different ways. Over the years, this development process intertwined the Fugo blade, conjunctival lymphatics, and surgical techniques.

In this part of the book, we will explore ocular applications of the Fugo blade in a variety of surgical situations related to the treatment of glaucoma. See Chapters 25 to 34 for surgical techniques in specific conditions.

Integrative and Integrated Glaucoma Surgery

In some situations, the possibility of surgical failure is high. To achieve the greatest chance for a successful conclusion, certain steps can be carried out with the Fugo blade that either prevent failure or allow for easy secondary correction. Here are some common combinations.

1. Transciliary filtration (TCF) is combined with microtrack filtration (MTF) into the anterior chamber (the Atwal balanced approach) to drain both the posterior and anterior chambers.

2. The TCF pit is undermined toward the anterior chamber, reaching close to it but not opening it. This thin barrier may be opened with an yttrium–aluminum–garnet (YAG) laser in case of a reduced outflow of aqueous with an abnormal rise in intra-ocular pressure.

3. Nonperforating glaucoma surgery combined with tissue thinning toward the angle for subsequent opening with a YAG laser.

4. Nonperforating glaucoma surgery combined with MTF or TCF, when the surgeon is not convinced of success with nonperforating glaucoma surgery.

5. Cyclodialysis combined with MTF or TCF.

Many more possibilities and iterations exist, depending on the situation. Local mitomycin drops 0.04% seven to eight times a day can be prescribed. These drops are kept in the refrigerator and prepared fresh every third day. The drops are continued for 15 days. In addition, the tracks created by a Fugo blade allow for placement of setons and valve tubing.

Summary

Currently, because of uncertainties and complications that arise with the surgical management of glaucoma, most physicians are interested in continuing medical management of glaucoma. Only when the situation worsens is surgery considered, and by then it may be too late for the patient.

No doubt, successful medical control of glaucoma is a relief to both patient and physician. But the medications, the repeat visits, and the continuous tests to keep the condition in check all add up a constant financial drain on the patient. But millions of patients cannot afford the luxury of medication, for psychological and financial reasons. A successful surgery is a blessing for rich and poor alike, a release from the daily worry of medication and from the continued drain on resources.

The Fugo blade glaucoma techniques described in this book are just the beginning. I can foresee great refinements coming. Those refinements may one day elevate the surgical management of glaucoma to the first line of treatment.

Suggested Reading

Allingham RR, Damji KF, Freedman S, Moroi SE. *Shields' textbook of glaucoma.* 5th ed. Philadelphia, Pa: Lippincott Williams & Wilkins 2004.

Conjunctival Lymphatics DALJIT SINGH and TAJ KIRMANI

A description of conjunctival lymphatics is important for this book, as some Fugo blade techniques for glaucoma are designed to minimize trauma to the lymphatics.

The lymphatics are certainly present under the conjunctiva, because their existence can be demonstrated. They must be present in the orbit too, even if they cannot be seen. If no lymphatics existed in these sites, what would happen to a subconjunctival hematoma or to a large retrobulbar hemorrhage, say, after retrobulbar injection? Extravasated blood may not re-enter the circulation through the venous capillaries; only in two ways can the blood return: quick return via lymphatics or a prolonged breakdown of the blood elements into basic elements, which are then absorbed. Venous capillaries cannot open up as lymphatics can.

The conjunctival lymphatics are orphan structures; they have not been adopted for study by most ophthalmologists, including glaucoma specialists. Key texts in the literature offer a narrow spectrum of views on ocular lymphatics, ranging from "the eye contains no lymphatics" to brief comments on ocular lymphatics, usually limited to fewer than a dozen sentences. Confusion stems from the fact that few have seen lymphatics. The ophthalmology community has a kind of "gut feeling" that they do not exist. The pathophysiology of ocular tissues is rarely if ever explained on the basis of the presence of lymphatics.

How can the eye manage fluid imbalance without the lymphatics? Consider the uveoscleral outflow that accounts for more than 50% of the aqueous outflow, and the leakage from the aqueous veins. Which system comes into play when filtration surgery is performed? Which system is to be blamed when a filtration operation fails? What produces large avascular blebs? These and many other questions can be answered if the presence and the function of the lymphatics is recognized.

We have studied lymphatics in trauma cases in the outpatient setting and in the operating room.

Conjunctival Lymphatics in the Outpatient Setting

The easiest way to study lymphatics is to observe the limbus through the high-power magnification of a slit-lamp microscope. The transparent lymphatics can be visualized, although they are hard to see at first. The definition is improved by the presence of pigment at the limbus. The lymphatics are more easily observed in dark-skinned people of all shades than in whites; because the white population generally lacks much pigment in the iris, its absence in the limbal area is to be expected. Acknowledging the presence of the lymphatics is the first step toward considering their role in the transport of aqueous in health and disease.

Raw lymphatics are frequently and easily recognized, once we know what they look like. These fairly large transparent structures run parallel to the limbus and give the conjunctiva a corrugated appearance (Fig. 25.1). The corrugated appearance is enhanced if the cornea is viewed under a slit-lamp.

The lymphatics at the limbus are fine channels running perpendicular to it. They are best visualized if some pigment is near the limbus. The general pattern is very apparent: vertical limbal channels flow into the

25

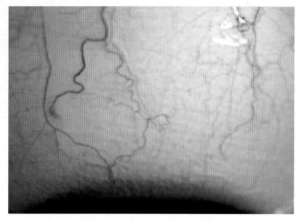

Figure 25.1. The raw lymphatics are visible as transparent channels running parallel to the limbus.

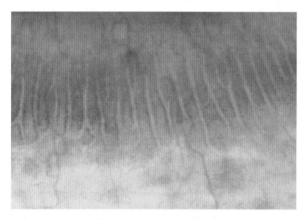

Figure 25.2. This image shows well-defined limbal lymphatics disappearing into the cornea at one end and merging with circularly running channels proximally.

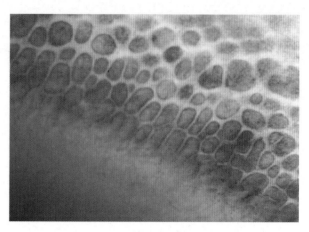

Figure 25.3. A network of lymphatics that has been outlined by the limbal pigment outside the transparent vessels. The finer channels close to the limbus run perpendicularly. Proximally they join each other and the wider circular channels.

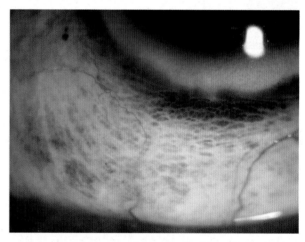

Figure 25.4. An extensive network of lymphatic channels at and around the limbus, reaching toward the fornix.

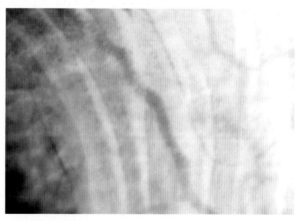

Figure 25.5. Rivulets of lymphatics are clearly outlined by the pigment around the limbus. The blood vessels appear pale where they are crossed anteriorly by the lymphatics.

the circular anastomosing channel network. The corneal ends of the limbal lymphatics seem to disappear and merge into a channel network in the cornea. See Figures 25.2 to 25.5 for examples.

Frequently finds blood appears in the lymphatics as a result of trauma, including surgical trauma. The pattern of blood-filled lymphatics is very different from the pattern of arteries and veins with which we are all familiar (Fig. 25.6).

Conjunctival Lymphatics in the Surgical Setting

In the surgical setting, lymphatics can be demonstrated by injecting trypan blue into the periphery of the cornea. The dye soon spreads to fill the lymphatic

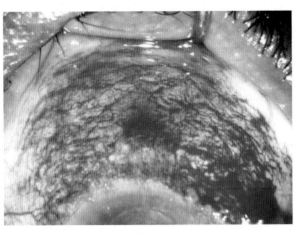

Figure 25.6. A surgical injury to a blood vessel at the 3 o'clock position starting to fill the lymphatics. In less than a minute, a large network of lymphatics became visible.

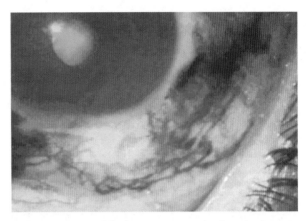

Figure 25.8. In failed surgery cases, the lymphatics are either absent or appear abnormal.

network. The network is extensive in every case, but the extent of the network that can be visualized varies from patient to patient. The radial lymphatic vessels close to the limbus are thinner than the network of circular vessels proximally. One or more channels arise from this system and disappear toward the fornices (Fig. 25.7).

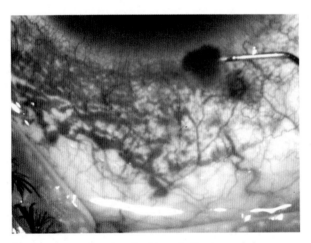

Figure 25.7. A network of lymphatic channels has become visible after injection of trypan blue into the periphery of the cornea.

In cases of failed glaucoma surgery, we have found that scarred areas do not display the lymphatics. Whatever type of surgery has been performed on the globe (e.g., strabismus, glaucoma, or retinal surgery) the lymphatics will be damaged at the incision and bipolar cautery sites. This is one good reason why tissues should be handled as little as possible in all kinds

of operations. Glaucoma surgery is doomed if attempts are made to produce a drainage track in a previously handled area (Fig. 25.8).

Relationship between Uveoscleral Outflow and Conjunctival Lymphatics

The literature is replete with information on uveoscleral outflow, but does not explain how and where this outflowing fluid is deposited. In one of our studies with trypan blue in a patient who had extensive scarring around the limbus, we found a startling connection between the sclera and subconjunctiva. Dye was injected into the sclera close to the limbus, traveled through the sclera, and appeared at multiple points around the limbus as blue blots and knots, indicating that the dye had traveled through some sort of channels inside the sclera. It also indicated that further connections of these blots were missing. However, when we looked at the conjunctiva proximal to the damaged area, we noticed that the conjunctival lymphatics had received the blue dye. We demonstrated this phenomenon in two more cases. How did an injection in the sclera fill the conjunctival lymphatics at such a distance? The only rational answer is that some form of three-dimensional network connects scleral lymphatics to the conjunctival network. And this raises another question: How does the uveoscleral outflow function? This scleroconjunctival connection suggests that not only mere diffusion but actual transport through normal existing channels may occur. Thus, uveoscleral-conjunctival outflow may be as much a secure closed channel transport system as the Schlemm canal-aqueous vein (Fig. 25.9).

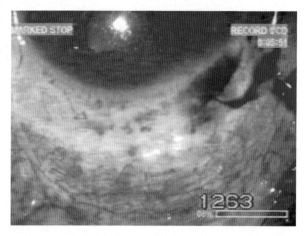

Figure 25.9. Extensive scarring appears around the limbus. Trypan blue injected near the damaged limbus has appeared in multiple blots along the limbus. But it has also filled up the proximal conjunctival lymphatics, proving the existence of channels directly connecting the scleroconjunctival system.

Summary

All evidence collected from our slit-lamp examinations and dye-injection studies indicates that an important three-dimensional lymphatic channel system exists under the conjunctiva and that it is connected to a similar scleral channel system. This lymphatic system is responsible for the drainage of normal outflowing aqueous. It can cope with the excessive fluid that drains after glaucoma filtration operations. Obstruction to free flow through the lymphatics results in the formation of blebs. Damage to the lymphatic system triggers subconjunctival fibrosis, which may become excessive and thereby jeopardize the successful outcome of a filtration operation. We believe that patients with glaucoma can be treated more successfully if the role of conjunctival lymphatics in aqueous drainage is taken into consideration when designing surgical techniques.

Suggested Reading

Bethke WC. A new clue to lymphatic drainage? *Rev Ophthalmol.* 2002;9:12.

Kent C. Revealed: the eye's lymphatic system. *Ophthalmol Manage.* 2002;6:114.

Singh D. Conjunctival lymphatic system. *J Cataract Refract Surg.* 2003;29:632–633.

Singh D, Singh RSJ, Singh K, et al. The conjunctival lymphatic system. *Ann Ophthalmol.* 2003;3:99–104.

Nonperforating Glaucoma Surgery DALJIT SINGH

To avoid complications of trabeculectomy, such as hypotony, flat anterior chamber, and choroidal detachment, Fyodorov et al.[1] introduced an equivalent of deep sclerectomy. Kozov et al.[2] proposed a similar operation plus a collagen drain to improve external filtration. In 1991, Stegmann[3] proposed viscocanalostomy, which encompassed the injection of hyaluronic acid in both ends of the unroofed Schlemm canal. Since then numerous studies have been done, and nonperforating glaucoma surgery has become an important surgical technique for controlling glaucoma.

Nonperforating glaucoma surgery (NPGS) is done under the highest magnification of the microscope. A steep learning curve to performing the surgery exists. Currently, all nonperforating procedures which does not allow the blade to enter the eye are guarded. Two scleral flaps are fashioned, the deeper of which is removed to expose the Schlemm canal to remove its lateral wall. The dissection is carried forward so that only the Descemet membrane separates the anterior chamber from the external drainage chamber.

My colleagues and I first performed nonperforating surgery with the Fugo blade on a 30-year-old woman who was 8 months pregnant. She had high myopia and pseudophakia, and her intra-ocular pressure was uncontrolled at 38 mm Hg. Surgical and postoperative complications were to be avoided at all costs.

The surgery was done with an 8X operating loupe (Zeiss) and illuminated with the operating microscope. The conjunctiva was detached from the limbus. The limbal tissue over the Schlemm canal was slowly ablated with a 600-μm Fugo blade tip until a fluid ooze was seen.

The conjunctiva was then sutured back in place. Five years later, the patient retains a thin bleb, and her intra-ocular pressure is 14 mm Hg. Figure 26.1 is a three-dimensional image of the patient's present condition.

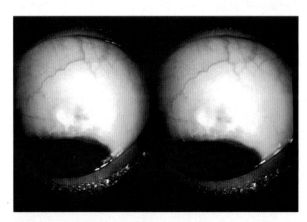

Figure 26.1. Three-dimensional image of an NPGS patient 5 years after surgery. The patient retains a thin bleb, and her intra-ocular pressure was reduced by more than 50% after surgery.

Since performing this procedure we have done numerous nonperforating operations in selected cases. Our surgical technique involves opening the Schlemm canal to the tissues under the conjunctiva. Success depends on the outflowing aqueous making its way to the subconjunctival drainage system. The following cases show how Fugo blade ablation can remove tissue to reach the desired depths accurately. This can be done without manual dissection, which requires high magnification.

CASE STUDIES

Case 1: Blunt Trauma with Lens Subluxation

A 23-year-old patient presented several days after suffering a blunt injury that caused subluxation of the lens and an intra-ocular pressure >50 mm Hg (Fig. 26.2).

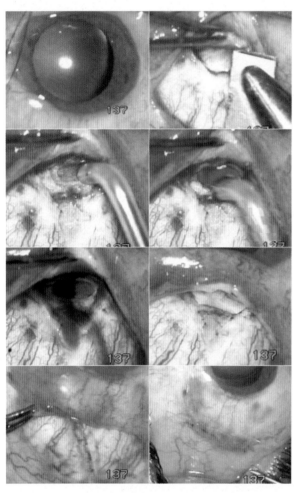

Figure 26.2. Trauma with lens subluxation (Case 1). A limbal-based conjunctival flap under which a triangular scleral flap reaches the limbus is seen. Ablation of limbus with a 600-μm Fugo blade tip opens the Schlemm canal. Aqueous movement is confirmed with a drop of trypan blue, the apex of the scleral flap is cut, the subconjunctival tissues are hydrated, and tenon capsule and conjunctiva are sutured separately.

Surgical Technique

1. Under a limbus-based flap, make a triangular scleral flap that exposes the limbal area.

2. Pass a 600-μm Fugo blade tip, set at low power and high intensity, lightly over the expected site of the Schlemm canal.

3. After a few passes of the Fugo blade, the outer wall of the Schlemm canal is breached, as indicated by aqueous oozing. A drop of trypan blue will be washed away, proving aqueous flow.

4. Remove part of the scleral flap. Hydrate the tenon capsule with saline before suturing it and the conjunctiva in separate layers.

Case 2: Uveitis and Glaucoma

A 40-year-old patient suffered chronic uveitis and secondary glaucoma that remained uncontrolled with medication (Fig. 26.3).

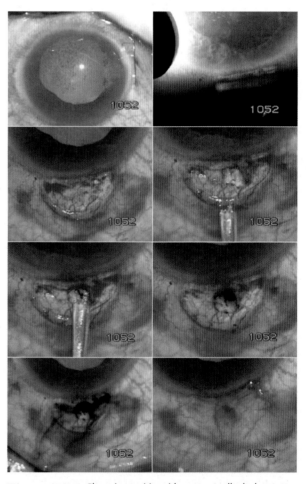

Figure 26.3. Chronic uveitis with uncontrolled glaucoma (Case 2). A fornix-based conjunctival flap is seen. Ablation of the limbus removes the lateral wall of the Schlemm canal. The aqueous flow is confirmed with the injection of trypan blue and the conjunctival flap is sutured.

26

Surgical Technique

1. Transilluminate the limbal area to judge the location of the angle and the Schlemm canal.

2. Make a 5-mm fornix-based flap to expose the limbal area.

3. Perform ablation by sweeping a 600-μm Fugo blade tip from the limbus upward until the aqueous flows from the Schlemm canal. Confirm aqueous flow with a drop of trypan blue.

4. Suture the conjunctival flap back in place.

Case 3: Open-Angle Glaucoma

To treat a patient with open-angle glaucoma, we used a spatulate form of the Fugo blade tip to do open ablation of the lateral wall of the Schlemm canal (Fig. 26.4), as in Case 2. Minimal dissection was required in this case. This case demonstrates how the Fugo blade can remove tissue without burning or charring.

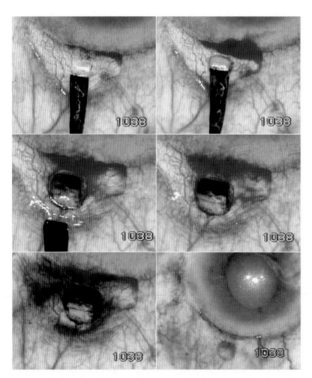

Figure 26.4. Open-angle glaucoma (Case 3). The lateral wall of the Schlemm canal is removed without making a scleral flap. The aqueous movement is confirmed with the injection of trypan blue, and the conjunctiva is sutured back.

Nonperforating Filtration Combined with Microtrack Filtration or Transciliary Filtration

If the aqueous ooze in NPGS appears less than satisfactory, or in the judgment of the surgeon the eye needs greater outflow of the aqueous, additional filtration routes can be added.

The limbus anterior to the nonperforating track can be undermined with a 600-μm Fugo blade tip, stopping just short of entering the anterior chamber. Creating this filtration area allows for filtration enhancement if necessary, by creating an opening using an yttrium–aluminum–garnet (YAG) laser. Or a track can be made right then and there with a 100-μm Fugo blade tip.

The area proximal to the area of nonperforating ooze can be thinned with a 600-m Fugo blade to reach the ciliary body. A 100-μm tip is used to make a track through the ciliary body into the posterior chamber (Fig. 26.5).

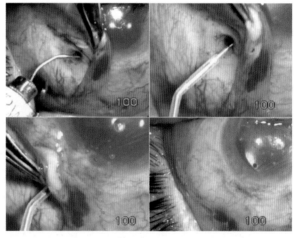

Figure 26.5. A fine cannula was introduced in the Schlemm canal, but fluid seepage was unsatisfactory. A 100-μm Fugo blade is directed toward the anterior chamber.

Summary

Nonperforating glaucoma surgery is not easy, and it has its complication. When manually removing fine tissues, perforations cannot be totally avoided. Successful NPGS depends on a number of factors, the most important being tissue reaction and scarring. However, the technique certainly has its merits. In some situations, any kind of perforating surgery, either in the anterior or the posterior chamber, is beset with risks. In these cases, NPGS is the best option. Use of the Fugo blade in NPGS allows the surgeon to ablate tissues in microscopic amounts in any standard or innovative manner to meet the needs of the case at hand.

Reference

1. Fyodorov SN, Kozlov VI, Timoshkina NT, et al. Nonpenetrating deep sclerectomy in open angle glaucoma. *Ophthalmosurgery*. 1990;3:52–55.

2. Kozlov VI, Bagarov SN, Anisimoba SY, et al. Nonpenetrating deep sclerectomy with collagen. *Ophthalmosurgery*. 1990;3:44–46.

3. Stegmann RC. Visco-canalostomy: a new surgical technique for open angle glaucoma. *An Inst Barraquer*. 1995;25:229–232.

Suggested Reading

Singh D, Fugo RJ. Glaucoma surgery techniques with the Fugo blade. In: Garg A, Fine IH, Pallikaris IG, et al., eds. *Innovative techniques in ophthalmology*. New Delhi, India: Jaypee, 2006:418–420.

Transconjunctival Transciliary Filtration (Singh Aqueous Bypass)

DALJIT SINGH,
KIRANJIT SINGH,
and C. THOMAS DOW

The goal of transconjunctival transciliary filtration (TCTCF) is to cause the posterior chamber fluid to drain under the subconjunctival space, without the need for dissection of any kind. An activated Fugo blade is directed through the conjunctiva, the tenon capsule, the sclera posterior to the scleral spur, and the pars plicata of the ciliary body to open the lateral wall of the posterior chamber. The track passes across the suprachoroidal space. The volume of the posterior chamber is merely one-fifth of the anterior chamber fluid. The inflow and outflow channels of aqueous are separated by the iris.

TCTCF is suitable for all patients in whom the posterior chamber anatomy is normal. This technique is eminently suitable in cases of phacomorphic glaucoma, either alone or immediately before lens surgery, acute congestive glaucoma, some cases of malignant glaucoma, and neovascular glaucoma. In eyes with scarred perilimbal conjunctiva resulting from earlier operations, you may find a healthy spot 1 or even 2 mm away from the limbus from where TCTCF can be performed.

TECHNIQUE

Anesthesia

Adequate local anesthesia includes a facial block and a choice between retrobulbar, peribulbar, and subconjunctival infiltration anesthesia. Mere surface anesthesia is not enough. After the injection, compress the eyeball for 5 minutes using a rubber ball to disperse the anesthetic agent in all directions. The patient will not feel pain during the procedure.

Surgical Technique

1. Separate the eyelids with a speculum. Make sure that the speculum is not stretching the fornix conjunctiva too much, as this may prevent proper execution of important surgical steps. The conjunctiva above the upper limbus or wherever surgery is to be done should be loose and mobile.

2. Visualize the posterior limit of the bluish surgical limbal area by pressing or stretching the conjunctiva. Mark it by pressing with the blunt side of a 1-mm diamond blade. Use the same blade to measure and mark 1 mm above the first mark. Now press the blunt side of a razor fragment on the sclera, parallel to the limbus. Maintain the pressure until a sufficient indentation (about 1 mm) is made on the conjunctiva and the sclera; the indentation acts as a guide when the conjunctiva is glided toward the limbus during the next step of surgery. A 1-mm diamond knife is the best measuring instrument. Performing TCTCF 1 mm behind the limbus site is not a hard-and-fast rule,

as variations are possible; for example, a variation is to be expected when the corneal diameter is smaller or larger than normal.

3. Use a blunt-edged nonmetallic tool to glide a fold of conjunctiva from the proximal to the limbal side, up to the marked indentation on the sclera. There, press the conjunctiva toward the sclera so that it cannot slip from underneath the pressing tool. An intentionally blunted diamond or sapphire knife is eminently suitable for this purpose, because it is nonmetallic.

4. Use a straight 300-μm naked ablation tip to open the posterior chamber. The naked tip produces a scleral-ciliary track that is wider than the blade itself. This helps you to be aware to some extent of what is happening under the tip. The tip remains functional as long the posterior chamber fluid has not been reached.

5. Place the naked 300-μm tip in direct proximity to the blunt diamond tool that controls the retracted conjunctiva. The Fugo blade is set at the highest energy level. The posterior chamber is approachable almost directly under the scleral indentation.

6. From where the entry point has been chosen (1 mm from the limbus), direct the ablating tip at about 70 to 90 degrees.

7. Activate the Fugo blade and insert it in small steps, taking it deeper with each step. After each little step, visualize the ablated pit for the depth.

8. When the sclera is ablated, the black ciliary body appears. Ablate the ciliary body slowly, in many steps. One last step takes the blade into the posterior chamber, and the fluid begins to drain. The aqueous comes out, sometimes mixed with black-pigmented specks. The aqueous fills the scleral–uveal track and makes any further ablation by the naked tip ineffective. (The track can be made in one complete step that takes the tip to the posterior chamber; however, it is wise to take these steps slowly.) When fluid surrounds the naked Fugo blade tip, its ablating power decreases automatically. The crystalline lens is in no danger because it is, in practical terms, located far from the surgical site.

9. Confirm the completion of transciliary filtration track formation by pushing air through it using a 24-gauge cannula. This can be achieved only if the conjunctiva retracting device is still in place after the aqueous has drained. Air flows into the anterior chamber after traveling under the iris and through the pupil.

10. Rinse the posterior chamber with saline if blood appears during the procedure.

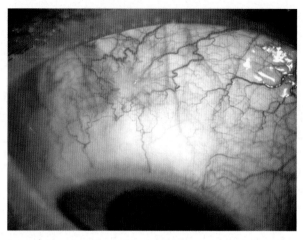

Figure 27.1. Mitomycin use causes avascularity in the area where it was applied during surgery.

11. If you use a 300-μm tip shielded with nonstick material, you will feel the resistance of the track wall as it is created. The ablation process is completely blocked from view as the tip fills the track. This not much of a problem, however, since the tip is repeatedly removed and the track observed as the track is being made.

12. Allow the conjunctiva to retract.

13. In selected cases, inject a drop of mitomycin 0.02% to 0.05% around the scleral opening with a thin cannula. The blebs resulting from filtration in these cases appear somewhat avascular. Mitomycin may help to prevent scarring in high-risk cases (Fig. 27.1).

14. The conjunctival hole resulting from the procedure is situated about 2 to 3 mm away from the scleral opening. It is secured with a suture or with fibrin glue. It can also be left alone to close naturally in a day or two.

In all cases with a shallow anterior chamber, the depth is seen to increase right after the posterior chamber begins to drain. In neovascular glaucoma cases, blood may begin to ooze from the angle of the anterior chamber. Nothing needs to be done; chances are that the blood in the anterior chamber will not compromise the ciliary body opening because the blood will collect in the lower part of the anterior chamber, while the filtering track is superior and behind the iris.

Postoperative Management

Worn off, remove the eye patch. Instruct the patient to instill topical steroid-antibiotic drops six to eight times during the day for 3 weeks. The patient should gradually decrease the drops over the next month. Use an antibiotic–steroid ointment at bedtime.

Examine the eye for the depth of the anterior chamber and the condition of the filtration area and the surrounding bleb. Examine the eye every week for a month. Beyond that, follow-up is determined by the individual needs of the patient.

The filtration area is prone to all the normal reactions of the subconjunctival area, the tenon capsule, and the scleral and ciliary body tissues surrounding the filtration track. However, the TCTCF technique causes very little tissue reaction.

CASE STUDIES

The utility of TCTCF is illustrated by the following diverse examples.

Case 1: Congestive Glaucoma

A 52-year-old patient had acute congestive glaucoma. The intra-ocular pressure (IOP) was above 50 mm Hg. The anterior chamber was very shallow and the cornea was edematous. The IOP could not be reduced with local or systemic medication. Surgery was recommended and performed as described below (Fig. 27.2).

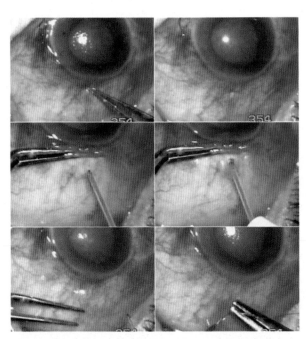

Figure 27.2. TCTCF in a case of acute congestive glaucoma (Case 1). A scleral depression is made with the tip of a forceps. The conjunctiva is pulled down beyond the depression using a plain forceps. A TCTCF track is made with a 300-μm tip. A bleb arises. The conjunctival hole is closed with a suture.

The tip of a forceps was pressed at the point of intended entry through the sclera. The pressure created a pit in the sclera that was visible through the conjunctiva. The conjunctiva was then slid down with a plane forceps. A 300-μm Fugo blade tip shielded with nonstick material was used to effect TCTCF. During the process of making the filtration track, the tip was not allowed to touch the metallic forceps. Once the fluid drainage was started, the surgery was complete. The conjunctival hole was closed with a suture. Postoperative recovery was uneventful (Fig. 27.3).

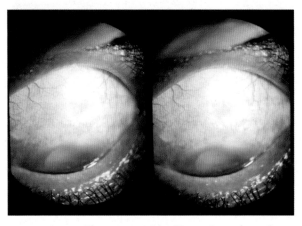

Figure 27.3. The same patient (Case 1) 15 days after surgery. The bleb is well formed and the anterior chamber is now normal.

Cases 2 and 3: Phacomorphic Glaucoma

In case 2, a 65-year-old patient had had acute phacomorphic glaucoma for 1 week. The IOP was above 50 mm Hg. The patient's pain was a major concern, as was the restoration of vision. Two possible avenues existed for treatment: either one-stage surgery for glaucoma and cataract, or control of the IOP as the first stage. We chose the latter. TCTCF surgery was performed as usual. The operation was considered satisfactory, as fluid mixed with some pigment drained out. The movement of the fluid was confirmed by putting a drop of trypan blue on the conjunctival hole (Fig. 27.4). One suture was applied to it. The recovery was uneventful (Fig. 27.5).

In a very similar case (Case 3), photographs taken before surgery and 3 days and 40 days after surgery show profound deepening of the anterior chamber. This could not happen without considerable shrinkage in the volume of the intumescent cataract (Fig. 27.6).

This case brings up the question of the relationship between phacomorphic glaucoma and intumescence

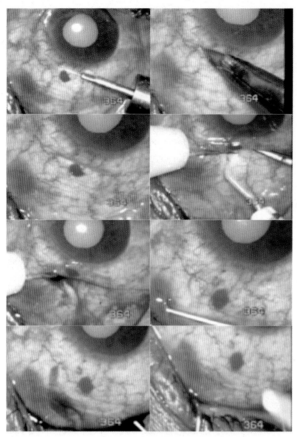

Figure 27.4. A case of phacomorphic glaucoma (Case 2). Successful TCTCF brings out some pigment and blood. Trypan blue dropped in the conjunctival opening flows away with the aqueous stream. The opening is closed with a suture.

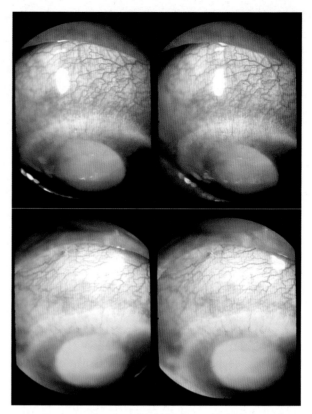

Figure 27.5. The same patient (Case 2), before and 3 hours after surgery, in three-dimensional imaging. The depth of the anterior chamber has considerably improved.

of the cataract. The attack of glaucoma no doubt results from angle closure. As the IOP rises, more aqueous enters the cataractous lens by hydrostatic pressure and increases its volume. This further increases the severity of obstruction, and thus begins a vicious circle. When the IOP falls, the fluid moves out of the cataract and the anterior chamber depth increases.

Case 4: Phthisis Bulbi and Staphylomas

A 20-year-old female patient had phthisis bulbi in one eye and extensive ciliary staphylomas, a deep anterior chamber, occlusion pupillae, and an IOP of 32 mm Hg in the second eye. Ultrasounic B mode (UBM) showed a voluminous space behind the iris produced as a result of thinning and stretching of the ciliary body. The sclera was nearly nonexistent in the staphyloma areas. Surprisingly, the patient had good all-around light projection. Any kind of standard filtration pro-

cedure was unthinkable. The entire anatomy of the anterior segment was disturbed, which made operations like trabeculectomy, nonperforating filtration, viscocanalostomy, and glaucoma valve procedures nearly impossible to perform. Over the preceding 2 years, the patient's search for control of her IOP was fruitless because the pressure could not be controlled with medication and surgery was never suggested.

Judging from our earlier experience with three similar cases, we believed that TCTCF could resolve the patient's glaucoma, and in fact the surgery was very simple. The freely mobile conjunctiva was glided down over the staphyloma at the 12 o'clock position. A 300-μm Fugo blade tip was used. The first light touch crossed the conjunctiva; the second light touched ablated the uveal tissue, and that released the aqueous fluid. The conjunctiva was slid back to its original position and a suture was applied to the conjunctival opening. The surgery produced a delicate extensive bleb over the surface of the sclera. The chances for the survival of this bleb are high, since the surgery was atraumatic and there were no tenon capsule or sclera to react to surgery and close the track (Fig. 27.7).

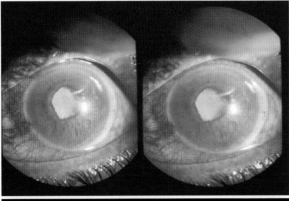

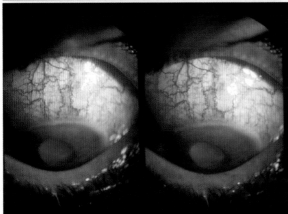

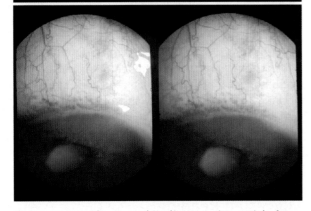

Figure 27.6. Phacomorphic glaucoma (Case 3) before surgery and 4 days and 40 days after surgery. The depth of the anterior chamber has increased. The congestion is gone.

Blebs after Transconjunctival Transciliary Filtration

The most striking thing about the blebs in the first 1 or 2 days after surgery is the remarkable similarity of their appearance. Most cases look alike in the first few days. The blebs are well formed and spread out diffusely. The most raised area of the conjunctiva lies over the scleral end of the filtration track. From this central

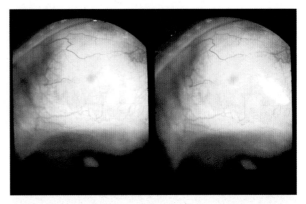

Figure 27.7. TCTCF in a case of ciliary staphyloma (Case 4), 1 day after surgery. A totally transparent conjunctiva (visible in three dimensions) is lifted by the outward flow of the aqueous.

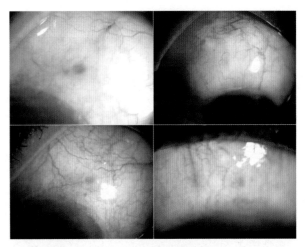

Figure 27.8. Examples of blebs that are less than 1 week old. The blebs are shallow and extensive.

point, the aqueous fluid drains diffusely. The appearance changes over time. In the coming days, the bleb becomes flatter as the filtration volume settles down according to the facility/resistance from the subconjunctival tissues, including the lymphatics (Fig. 27.8). They might flatten out yet remain effective (Fig. 27.9). The flattening appears quite natural since no obstruction from tissue reaction is formed and fluid is carried away by the lymphatics. It is not surprising to see a barely visible but fully functional bleb in an eye that had an IOP above 50 mm Hg before surgery.

Postoperative Management

The dressing is removed as soon as the effect of local anesthesia has worn off. The usual finding is a normal anterior chamber and a raised extensive bleb. The patient goes home with steroid antibiotic drops to be

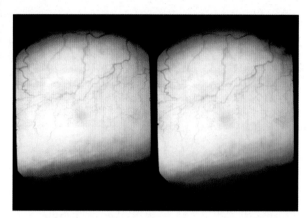

Figure 27.9. A TCTCF bleb, 2 months after surgery, in three dimensions. The bleb is barely raised from the surface, but is functional. The conjunctiva show a normal transparent gossamerlike appearance. The IOP is 15 mm Hg, down from 51 mm Hg before surgery.

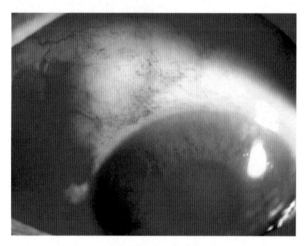

Figure 27.10. A postoperative blood ooze that originated either from the area of filtration or from the angle of the anterior chamber.

instilled seven to eight times a day and an antibiotic–steroid ointment for bedtime.

An occasional adverse finding is a blood ooze (Fig. 27.10). This is of no great concern, however, as the blood settles and absorbs spontaneously and does not interfere with the filtration track, which is far removed from the site, on the back of the iris.

Summary

Transconjunctival transciliary filtration has some merit in the treatment of glaucoma. A conjunctival flap is unnecessary, as is interference with the tenon capsule and sclera. The route of tissue ablation to reach the posterior chamber is straight and does not damage adjacent tissues. This technique then becomes the minimally traumatic way to perform major filtration surgery. The key is to enter the sclera at the right point and to move in the right direction toward the posterior chamber. If suitable precautions are taken, the crystalline lens is in no danger. The Fugo blade tip becomes inactivated when it reaches the fluid in the posterior chamber.

In aphakic and pseudophakic pupillary block, TCTCF is very effective. UBM findings provide useful information for better placement and direction of the Fugo blade ablating tip. Repeat operation is easy and may be performed at the original site or at an adjacent site. Going through the tenon capsule as in TCTCF minimizes the chances of a tenon cyst formation.

In the future, a highly flexible miniature fiberoptic light and camera may be mounted on the Fugo blade tip to provide a high-quality high-magnification view of the ablation pit. Also, an electronic echo function may be incorporated in the ablating tip to show the precise shortest path in which the tip should be moved to cross the ciliary tissue to reach the fluid chamber.

Suggested Reading

Garg A, Fine H, Pallikaris IG, Chang DF, Tsuneoka H, Bovet JJ, eds. *Innovative techniques in ophthalmology*. New Delhi, India: Jaypee, 2006:414.

Atwal's Balanced Approach for Glaucoma Filtration

EPHRAIM SINGH ATWAL
and AMARJIT SINGH ATWAL

28

The objective of this chapter is to present a filtration procedure capable of achieving pressure stability without the need for medication or daily monitoring, while minimizing the incidence of complications such as shallow anterior chamber, hyphema, hypotony, and the concomitant use of antimetabolites. In our attempts to maintain the technical ease of the Singh filtration procedure and minimizing the incidence of complications and failure, the best outcome occurred when combining transciliary filtration (TCF) and microtrabeculectomy into one procedure while using Fugo blade technology. Previous attempts at microtrabeculectomy with Holmium lasers and minishunts were riddled with complications such as a flat or shallow chamber. When combining TCF with microtrabeculectomy, microfiltration is achieved with revolutionary success and no impediments.

The key to the procedure is that aqueous drainage from the posterior chamber of the eye changes the force vector dynamics of the aqueous such that minimal force pushes the iris forward, thus preventing an anterior chamber collapse. Furthermore, the TCF pore is placed behind the iris root through the pars plicata. As the eye pressure increases, the pars plicata is stretched, thereby opening the TCF pore and increasing aqueous flow. When the intra-ocular pressure (IOP) decreases, the pars plicata tissue becomes flaccid and partially collapses over the TCF ostomy opening, thereby slowing aqueous outflow. Thus, the posterior chamber TCF ostomy acts as an autoregulatory valve.

Our approach (the Atwal balanced approach, or ABA) can be performed in patients with phakia or pseudophakia. The best results were obtained with phaco-emulsification and subsequent ABA filtration in a combined procedure; this combination comprised the bulk of our study.

The benefits of finding a procedure that can effectively eliminate the need for glaucoma medications are numerous. It is estimated that 25% of patients with glaucoma do not take their medications at all, and a large percentage do not adhere to their entire prescription regimen or do not follow their course of therapy properly. It has been suggested that this noncompliance is a leading cause of blindness from glaucoma. Eliminating medication entirely or getting ocular pressure under control greatly improves the prognosis. This is especially true in the enormous third world nations, where even the cheapest medication is often not affordable.

Reasons for noncompliance with topical medications for glaucoma are numerous and include cost, poor memory, difficulty with lifestyle, the patient "giving up," poor finger dexterity, difficulty in mobility to gain access to medication, low intellect, and depression. The incidence of glaucoma is age-related. As our population ages, the incidence of glaucoma increases. The cost of eye drops is rather substantial, and when patients are on multiple-drop therapy, the regimen becomes such an

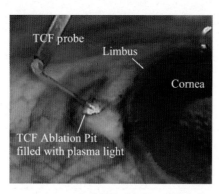

Figure 28.1. A standard TCF ablation pit is being created through sclera and pars plicata into the posterior chamber of the eye. Notice the light generated at the TCF ablation site by the Fugo blade plasma cloud. This ablation takes just seconds to perform.

encumbrance that they are often caught between paying for their eye drops or paying the rest of their bills. Such economic challenges along with issues of physical dexterity and other limitations present a major encumbrance for long-term compliance with an eye drop regimen. Glaucoma is the leading cause of blindness worldwide, with an incidence of 4.5 million patients per year.[1] For this reason, the World Health Organization has placed a major emphasis on a global effort to combat loss of vision caused by glaucoma.[1]

The ABA procedure is a modification of the U.S. Food and Drug Administration's (FDA) approved filtration procedure named after Dr. Daljit Singh of Amritsar, India, also called "Singh filtration" or "transciliary filtration" (TCF)[2,3] (Fig. 28.1). In this procedure, Dr. Singh used the eximer-laser–like qualities of the Fugo blade to ablate tissue with minimal energy (less than 3 W) while leaving pristine ablation incision walls.[4] TCF had been performed at our facility, and it was our opinion that TCF was successful in reducing eye pressure while eliminating flat anterior chambers because the aqueous fluid was drained from the posterior chamber of the eye, thereby relieving force vectors on the posterior surface of the iris. For this reason, it became clear that TCF was successful because it balanced the pressures between the posterior chamber and the anterior chamber better than the trabeculectomy procedure, which still suffers from flat anterior chambers. We modified the TCF procedure to create the ABA in an attempt to refine and improve the balance of pressure between the posterior and anterior chambers of the eye and achieve a higher and longer-term success rate.[3] The ABA procedure uses the standard TCF procedure followed by a Fugo blade ablation minitrabeculectomy/minitrabeculostomy into the anterior chamber angle, under a standard scleral flap. The entire surgical procedure takes less than 5 minutes and produces minimal tissue trauma. And because minimal tissue is traumatized, minimal eye inflammation is produced.

Materials and Methods

We evaluated whether the ABA procedure could provide IOPs equal to or lower than the those achieved when maximal medical therapy was indeed being practiced by patients. These patients had documented poor compliance during the previous year, with subsequent progression of glaucoma damage. Also all patients are non-compliant with drops at one time or another.

Patients were evaluated preoperatively and 1 day, 1 to 2 weeks, 4 to 6 weeks, 2 to 4 months, 5 to 7 months, and 8 to 12 months postoperatively. Surgical complications as well as postoperative complications were documented.

Statistical analysis was performed by obtaining p values. A test statistic was generated by comparing the group arithmetic mean divided by the sum of the group standard error values. The test statistic achieved was then plotted on a standard normal Z distribution curve, wherein a p value was calculated.

The ABA procedure was performed using the FDA-approved Fugo blade unit manufactured by Medisurg, Ltd. of Norristown, PA (Fig. 28.2). The Fugo blade is currently FDA-approved for capsulotomy, TCF for glaucoma, iridotomy formation for glaucoma, anterior chamber intra-ocular lenses, and the implantable contact lens. The Fugo blade is a low-powered monopolar electrosurgical unit that ablates tissue much like a mini-eximer laser rather than producing a cautery action.[4] The unit produces a 100-μm thick plasma cloud on a blunt hair-thin cutting filament (Fig. 28.3).

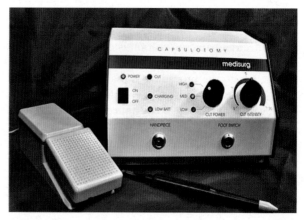

Figure 28.2. The Fugo blade unit consists of an electronic console, an ergonomic handpiece, and an activation foot switch.

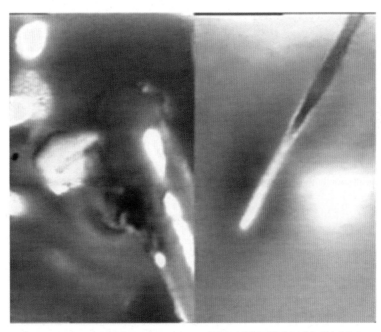

Figure 28.3. This image demonstrates an activated Fugo blade ablation tip. The tip is blunt and as thin as a human hair. The image on the left demonstrates light being emitted from the 100-μm thick plasma cloud. The image on the right filters out the light, thereby exposing the 100-μm thin plasma cloud that coats the blunt cutting filament. This plasma is nonarcing, but rather has a calm nature.

TECHNIQUE

Surgical Technique

1. Make a 600-μm-diameter ablation pit 1 to 2 mm behind the limbus until the darker ciliary body is seen (Fig. 28.4).
2. With the thin Fugo blade tip, enter the posterior chamber through the pars plicata. This creates a 200-μm ablation path through which aqueous percolates (Fig. 28.5).

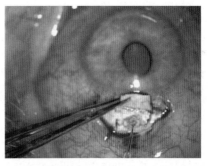

Figure 28.5. Fugo blade tip ablating through sclera and pars plicata into the posterior chamber.

3. At this stage, with the same thin Fugo tip, create a microtrabeculectomy anterior to the TCF from the base of the scleral flap and through the trabeculum in the anterior chamber (Fig. 28.6). Aqueous percolates much faster through the microtrabeculectomy site.
4. Then push the scleral flap back into position without sutures.
5. Suture back the conjunctival peritomy with two 10-0 nylon sutures or just cauterize at either end.
6. Patch the eye overnight.

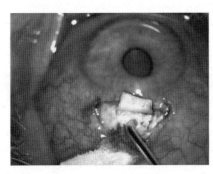

Figure 28.4. Creation of scleral ablation pit with activated Fugo blade tip.

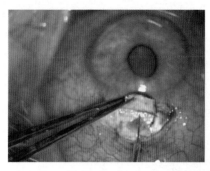

Figure 28.6. Fugo blade tip ablating through trabeculum into the anterior chamber.

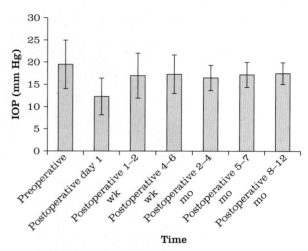

Figure 28.7. Average IOPs after ABA (arithmetic mean ±SD) preoperatively and at various intervals postoperatively.

Postoperative Management

Postoperative management is no different than that for cataract/intra-ocular lens procedures not using ABA.

Results

The mean (±SD) IOP on the first day after operation in the ABA group on no medical treatment was 12.3±4.12 mm Hg. An important clinical observation in this group was the lack of anterior chamber collapse. In several of the patients, there was mild shallowing of the anterior chamber; however, this was not significant enough to elicit peripheral anterior synechia or endothelial touch. All chambers had deepened by 1 week after surgery. In five patients, we had a small amount of anterior chamber blood that produced less than a 1-mm hyphema. This resolved with conservative therapy and without incidence. Spaeth et al.[5] demonstrated that trabeculectomy IOPs stabilized by 1 month after surgery. In actuality, the data from Spaeth et al. documented IOPs at 3 days and then at 1 month after surgery. Here, we document results 1 day, 1 to 2 weeks, 4 to 6 weeks, 2 to 4 months, 5 to 7 months, and 8 to 12 months after surgery (Fig. 28.7 and Table 28.1). We found that the ABA pressure stabilized at 1 to 2 weeks postoperatively. Our 1-to-2 week postoperative IOP mean was 17.0±5.06 mm Hg. When the Spaeth et al. data were compared with the present study, we found that there was no statistically significant difference between the primary glaucoma group treated with trabeculectomy in the Spaeth study at 1 year after surgery as compared with the ABA study at 8 to 12 months after surgery ($p > 0.05$). On the other hand, when we compared the primary glaucoma group and the secondary glaucoma group treated with trabeculectomy in the Spaeth study and the present ABA study, we found that the Spaeth study demonstrated a statistically signifi-

Table 28.1. Intra-ocular Pressures (mm Hg)[a]

Time	No. of Patients	Mean ±SD
Preoperative	139	19.5±5.47
Postoperative day 1	139	12.3±4.12
Postoperative 1–2 wk	137	17.0±5.06
Postoperative 4–6 wk	92	17.3±4.33
Postoperative 2–4 mo	98	16.5±2.83
Postoperative 5–7 mo	55	17.2±2.80
Postoperative 8–12 mo	53	17.5±2.43

[a]Data derived from the ABA study at various times during the study.

cantly higher 1-year IOP, with an arithmetic mean of 21.2±9.8 mm Hg ($p < 0.01$).

Complications in our study included five <1-mm hyphemas; these resolved with conservative therapy. In two eyes, small choroidal effusion occurred, which resolved spontaneously. Several patients had only minor anterior chamber shallowing, which resolved over the first postoperative week. During the course of the year, 9 of the 139 eyes needed topical eye drops added to their course of treatment in order to further reduce the IOP. To a large extent, these eye drops were added in eyes that had extremely advanced glaucomatous disc changes.

As with the Singh procedure, ABA places a precise TCF ablation pore through sclera into the posterior chamber of the eye. It should be noted that anatomic landmarks were initially used to locate the exact spot immediately behind the iris to ablate an ablation pore, although some may find it useful to locate the exact spot of the ablation site by using anterior chamber transillumination. The secret of TCF is that it decompresses aqueous from the posterior chamber of the eye through the pars plicata and the sclera. In this way, the force vectors are better equalized in the anterior and posterior chambers of the eye based on Bernoulli's principle of fluid dynamics. The idea of modifying TCF to create the ABA procedure was based on the observation that this balancing of pressure produced fewer complications, since aqueous force vectors were no longer directed exclusively at the TCF pore but were now divided and balanced between the TCF pore in the posterior chamber and the microtrabeculectomy in the anterior chamber. Therefore, it was hypothesized that an even more precise balancing of these pressures could potentially offer a higher success rate with a lower complication rate. For this reason, we decided to place the TCF pore immediately behind the iris under a standard trabeculectomy flap. The TCF pore ablation takes from 30 seconds to a minute to perform. Following the decompressive Fugo blade ablation ostomy into the posterior chamber of the eye, you take a standard 100-μm-diameter Fugo blade probe and position it at the base of the scleral flap. Then, you aim the ablation tip at the anterior chamber angle. You activate the Fugo blade and then perform a quick in-and-out maneuver to create a precise minitrabeculectomy ostomy into the anterior chamber. This procedure takes several seconds to perform.

After the TCF ablation into the posterior chamber, a fulminant ooze of aqueous is seen to exit through the TCF pore. Likewise, the minitrabeculectomy placed at the base of the scleral flap and into the anterior chamber angle produces fulminant flow from the anterior chamber of the eye. Thereby, ABA produces flow from both anterior and posterior chamber ostomy openings. This dual flow creates an ultimate balancing of pressures between the anterior and posterior chambers of the eye and produces pressure stabilization with little complication. Total surgical time is less than 5 minutes, and the procedure has been found to be minimally traumatic to the patient, largely because the size of the surgical site is so small. Unlike trabeculectomy, no sutures are used on the scleral flap.

The maximal ideal medical therapeutic baseline was found to be 19.5±5.5 mm Hg preoperatively. The IOP on postoperative day 1 was 12.3±4.12 mm Hg. This was comparable to the postoperative day 1 pressure in a standard trabeculectomy studies. For example, the classic study of Blondeau and Phelps demonstrated a postoperative day 1 trabeculectomy pressure of 12.1±11.6 mm Hg.[6] The standard deviation in the trabeculectomy in the study of Blondeau and Phelps

was higher because there was a much wider range of eye pressures in this group as compared with the ABA postoperative day 1 group. Sixty-eight percent of the Blondeau and Phelps group had an eye pressures from 0.6 to 23.8 mm Hg, whereas 68% of the ABA group had eye pressures from 8.1 to 16.5 mm Hg. Again, this demonstrates the control that is achievable when the pressures are balanced between the anterior and posterior chambers of the eye and substantially adds to the efficacy of the procedure. This demonstrates much higher hypotony in the trabeculectomy study group. The significance of the mean IOPs on postoperative day 1—12.2 mm Hg in the Blondeau and Phelps group versus 12.3 mm Hg in the ABA group—demonstrates a comparable overall effect of the procedures. However, a closer look at the standard deviation demonstrates that more precise control is achievable with the ABA procedure, which may be a factor in the relatively low incidence of postoperative complications. Unlike the Scheie procedure, which has been reported[5] to have over a 50% flattening of the anterior chamber, not a single patient who underwent ABA had a flat anterior chamber after the procedure—139 prospective cases in this study. At the time of writing, we have yet to experience a flat anterior chamber with either pure TCF or the ABA procedure. It should be noted that only one case of a flat anterior chamber after TCF has been reported in large TCF series being conducted by Thomas Dow, Daljit Singh, and Richard Fugo (personal correspondence).

Postoperative stabilization of the IOP was shown to occur between 1 and 2 weeks postoperatively using the ABA procedure. This is essentially comparable to the works of Blondeau and Phelps[6] as well as the classic work of Spaeth et al.,[5] in which it was demonstrated that stabilization of IOP occurred between 1 and 3 months postoperatively.

The preoperative ABA data were then compared with the postoperative ABA data, including data for 1 to 2 weeks, 4 to 6 weeks, 2 to 4 months, 5 to 7 months, and 8 to 12 months postoperatively. Statistical analysis for all ABA data groups was performed using p values by correlating the test statistic to the corresponding Z distribution curve. This demonstrated that there was no statistical significance ($p > 0.05$) between the 1-to-2-week, the 4-to-6-week the 2-to-4-month, the 5-to-7-month, and the 8-to-12-month postoperative ABA data. This essentially agrees with published trabeculectomy and thermosclerostomy results.[6] The 8-to-12-month data demonstrated a mean IOP of 17.5±2.4 mm Hg. This was comparable to the 1-year trabeculectomy data of Blondeau and Phelps, which was 17.1±7.4 mm Hg. The ABA results also corresponded well with the 1-year postoperative

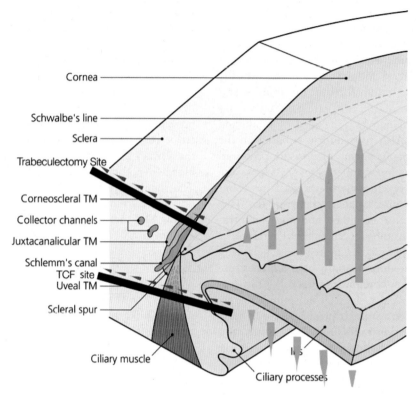

Figure 28.8. By performing trabeculectomy with TCF, we balance out the opposing forces, and obtain the benefits of both procedures.

results of the Spaeth et al. group with primary glaucoma treatment with trabeculectomy, which was 16.1 ± 4.5 mm Hg. In both cases, the ABA data were statistically compared using p values correlating the test statistic to the corresponding Z distribution chart for 1-year data. The IOPs were found to be equivocal and statistically nonsignificant ($p >0.05$). It should be emphasized, however, that both trabeculectomy studies demonstrated significantly higher standard deviations; therefore, there was a subsequent increase in variability on the high side and the low side for both trabeculectomy groups. This results in more patients with elevated IOPs as well as more hypotony. We believe that the lower standard deviation for ABA is based on the balanced-pressure dynamics established between the anterior and posterior chambers due to the dual filtration system created during the ABA procedure.

The preoperative maximal ideal medical therapeutic baseline and standard deviation for the ABA procedure was compared with all of the postoperative categories that were tabulated for the ABA group. It was found that the values for all of the postoperative groups were statistically lower than the preoperative groups. Deriving these results from our data pool was based mainly on the relatively large sample size as well as the low standard deviations that were achieved. It should

be emphasized that this demonstrates that the ABA procedure produced consistently lower eye pressures than were achieved by preoperative maximum medical therapy, which was strictly enforced preoperatively. In some cases, eye pressures may drop after cataract surgery for reasons such as low-grade iritis. However, a consistent drop of IOP after ABA with such tight standard deviation values is most unlikely as a secondary consequence of cataract surgery, especially with the relatively large sample size that was evaluated. Therefore, it is almost certain that the positive effects experienced and measured statistically are based on the positive effects of the pressure balances achieved with the ABA procedure (Fig. 28.8). Nine of the 139 patients had topical medications instituted during the course of a 1-year follow-up. This represents only 6.5% of the total test group; 3 of the patients had two eye drops added, and the remaining 6 had one eye drop added. It is likely that these patients will continue on the path of noncompliance. If significant progression in glaucoma is observed in this eye drop group, the patients will probably be considered for a repeat ABA procedure based on therapeutic noncompliance.

A point of interest to practitioners is the through-and-through ostomy created with the ABA procedure. One might hypothesize that such through-and-through openings would produce intractable hypotony. This is not the case. As a matter of fact, as we explained with the 1-day postoperative data, we have mean values comparable to those obtained with trabeculectomy; however, less hypotony was measured based on the lower standard deviation in the ABA study.[6]

The TCF ostomy is an opening through the pars plicata of the eye. As the eye pressure increases, the eye becomes tense, thereby causing stretching of the tissue, which results in the TCF pore opening more widely and allowing more aqueous fluid to escape. As the eye pressure decreases, the eye wall becomes more flaccid and the dynamics of the pars plicata come into play. The pars plicata actually droops or herniates into the ostomy opening, thereby reducing the aperture size of the ABA/TCF pore. Therefore, these ablation pores are not static, as would be seen if the eyeball were fabricated from material such as plastic. Rather, the eyeball is living tissue that has dynamics based on the physiologic characteristics of the eye, thereby producing the autoregulatory mechanism that controls and regulates the outflow of aqueous fluid. This effect is demonstrated in our postoperative day 1 data, which shows mean IOPs comparable to those for trabeculectomy studies, but with a lower standard deviation and therefore more IOP stability with less hypotony.[6] This autoregulatory mechanism has been substantiated by Dr. Steven Gross, a veterinary ophthalmologist in Philadelphia. Gross has performed numerous TCF procedures in dogs with glaucoma. (Dogs have much thicker ciliary bodies than humans.) Gross places a 600-μm pore through the ciliary body and has not reported hypotony as a significant problem in his surgeries because of the herniation of the ciliary body into the 600-μm TCF pore when the IOP decreases.

It should be emphasized that a very delicate handling of the conjunctiva is imperative in order to minimize trauma to the conjunctiva. In this way, the conjunctiva remains healthy and effective in aqueous removal into the circulatory system. Therefore, the postoperative bleb will not be bullous, but rather will be low and smooth, thereby creating an excellent barrier to infection and a nontraumatized, comfortable bleb that may work efficiently for many years.

Two eyes in our study group had small choroidal effusions, which resolved spontaneously. Five had a 10 to 15% hyphema, which also resolved without consequence. In retrospect, some patients abuse aspirin and nonsteroidal anti-inflammatory drugs (or NSAIDs) for pain such as arthritis. Furthermore, many popular homeopathic herbs and remedies—such as fish oil, flax oil, ginkgo, green tea, beta carotene, vitamin A, vitamin C, vitamin E, and garlic—reduce blood coagulation.

Three filters were complete failures (i.e., no bleb formation with IOP elevation >25 mm Hg) in eyes that underwent ABA for uncontrolled pressure under maximum medical therapy.

Simplicity is the ABA procedure's true asset. We have been able to eliminate or minimize medications for the majority of our patients using a procedure that effectively takes only minutes to perform and is truly cost-effective.

Summary

Our study provides a step-by-step outline on how the ABA procedure is performed and demonstrates statistically the safety and efficacy of the ABA procedure. This prospective study demonstrates that a procedure that takes <5 minutes and has low postoperative complications has the ability to lower the IOP more than maximum medical therapy. The ABA procedure also demonstrates eye pressure control that is comparable to that achieved with trabeculectomy. The difference between ABA and trabeculectomy is that the ABA procedure can be performed much more quickly, has relatively few side effects, and has a lower IOP standard deviation than has been cited in classic trabeculectomy studies. The basis of this excellent eye pressure control, low postoperative complication rate, and lower standard deviation in eye pressure is the precise balancing of IOP forces between the anterior and posterior chambers of the eye while achieving an overall lower IOP. For these reasons, we believe that the ABA procedure is a realistic candidate for the management of glaucoma worldwide.

References

1. World Health Organization. Socio economic aspects of blindness and visual impairment. Geneva, Switzerland: World Health Organization. Accessed January 9, 2007, at http://www.who.int/blindness/economy/en.
2. Singh D, Singh K. Transciliary filtration using the Fugo blade. *Ann Ophthalmol.* 2002;34:183–187.
3. Atwal A. "Atwal's balanced approach" for glaucoma filtration surgery presented. *Ocular Surg News.* 2005;19: 64–66.
4. Fine IH, Hoffman RS, Packer M. Highlights of the 2002 ASCRS Symposium, Part I. *Eyeworld.* 2002;7:38.
5. Spaeth GL, Joseph NH, Fernandes E. Trabeculectomy: a reevaluation after three years and a comparison with Scheie's procedure. *Trans Am Acad Ophthalmol Otolaryngol* 1975;79:349–361.
6. Blondeau P, Phelps CD. Trabeculectomy vs thermosclerostomy: a randomized prospective clinical trial. *Arch Ophthalmol.* 1981;99:810–816.

29 Ab Interno Pretenon Filtration DALJIT SINGH and KIRANJIT SINGH

Because the tenon capsule is a reactive tissue and contributes to filtration failure as a result of the formation of scarring, tenon cysts, or both, it is logical to avoid this tissue in the course of glaucoma surgery. The tenon capsule is firmly attached to the limbal connective tissue about 0.5 to 1 mm behind the insertion of the conjunctiva. This creates a potential pretenon space between the anterior conjunctiva and the limbal connective tissue. The Fugo blade makes it possible to use this space to create a filtering track, with the aim of minimizing tenon capsule involvement.

A track is made from the pretrabecular cornea to the distal pretenon potential subconjunctival space. As a primary procedure, it can be applied in all cases of glaucoma with moderate or deep anterior chambers, or in which at least the anterior chamber can be deepened during surgery. Peripheral iridectomy is mandatory. It is useful for cases in which the perilimbal area has been extensively damaged or fibrosed and any attempt to make a conjunctival flap has little chance of success. The only thing required is a virgin area of limbal and perilimbal conjunctiva, so that the outflowing aqueous can drain into the conjunctival lymphatics. The greater the intact virgin conjunctiva, the more the draining lymphatics can absorb the fluid load. Ultimately, it is the volume of the draining aqueous fluid that determines the final intra-ocular pressure. If the flow from inside is unimpeded, then resistance from the subconjunctival tissues and the carrying capacity of the lymphatics determine the level of success.

A number of specific factors affect the successful outcome of ab interno pretenon filtration, as discussed below.

First, the inner openings must be patent. This means the presence of no iris tissue, no pigment, no blood, no lens matter, no vitreous, no scar formation, no regrowth of endothelium over the site of the opening, and no edema of the cornea around the hole. The size of the opening should be adequate, but what constitutes "adequate size" is difficult to measure. The opening should be large enough to create fluid pressure sufficient to overcome subconjunctival resistance and allow for proper drainage, yet does not result in hypotony.

Second, the track is not closed, minimized, or compromised by any of the factors listed above.

Third, the fluid should not be dammed by byproducts of tissue reaction. To some extent this is natural and perhaps unavoidable. In order to drain, the outflowing aqueous has to negotiate as interstitial fluid through the reactive connective tissue to get into the lymphatic network of the conjunctiva, which is surrounded by the same connective tissue.

4.Fourth, post operative reactivity of the tenon connective tissue may have an effect. No hard-and-fast division between the subconjunctival connective tissue and the tenon capsule exists. A closure of the external opening of the filtering track may be simple scarring, which may or may not also extend inside the track, or it may be in the form of a raised dome sitting over the external opening. The size of this dome, or the so-called tenon cyst, varies. The thickness of the tenon cyst wall also varies from an initial thin wall that can be breached by pressing the eyeball to being so thick that you could call it "sclerification." High-risk cases include young eyes with a thick tenon capsule, trachomatous conjunctiva with pannus formation and fornix shrinkage, prolonged treatment with local antiglaucoma medication, and previously failed surgery.

Fifth, if mitomycin must be used in ab interno filtration, it has to be delivered beneath the conjunctiva, either before making the filtration or afterward. No optimal regimen of mitomycin application has been determined. For pretrack application, it should be injected under the conjunctiva close to the limbus where the track will be made. The optimal concentration and time must be determined by the surgeon. Afterward, it is thoroughly diluted and washed with lactated Ringer solution, which has an acidic pH and is good for this purpose. For posttrack application, the anterior chamber should first be blocked with sodium hyaluronate, so that no mitomycin enters it. At the end of the application, mitomycin is flushed from beneath the conjunctiva by copious irrigation in the anterior chamber. The fluid should come out of the initial opening that was made close to the limbus. Although we do not have enough experience to recommend precisely how to use mitomycin, we do believe its use should be limited to high-risk cases.

Finally, too many variables exist in any kind of filtration surgery. Ab interno filtration reduces the number of variables, especially with regard to tissue dissection, cauterization, application of mitomycin, and suturing. Some factors remain unresolved: exact entry and exit points, dimension of the filtering track, and tissue response to the draining aqueous.

TECHNIQUE

Anesthesia

Administer a facial block. Balloon the conjunctiva with lignocaine with adrenaline and apply a pressure bandage for 5 minutes. To avoid subconjunctival bleeding, open the conjunctiva with a 100-μm Fugo blade tip and inject the anesthetic fluid with a cannula.

Surgical Technique

1. Use a 100-μm Fugo blade to puncture the conjunctiva close to the limbus at the 11 o'clock position.

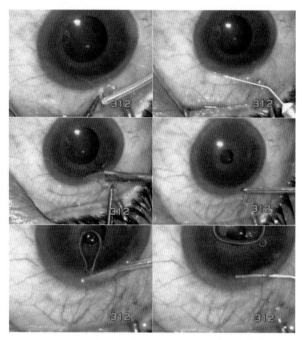

Figure 29.1. A 100-μm Fugo blade tip makes an opening in the conjunctiva close to the limbus. A 30-gauge cannula is routed beneath the distal pretenon conjunctiva and raises it by injecting sodium hyaluronate. A pocket incision is made in the cornea. A 300-μm tip is passed into the anterior chamber and is activated after touching the peripheral iris. An iridectomy is performed and becomes visible when the viscous agent is injected to deepen the anterior chamber.

2. Pass s curved 30-gauge cannula through this opening, and push it to negotiate the most distal, pretenon potential subconjunctival space up to the 1 o'clock position. Then balloon this track with sodium hyaluronate 1.4% or, preferably, 1.8% (Fig. 29.1).

3. Make a 1.5-mm-wide, deep pocket incision in the clear cornea. Make the incision obliquely so as to allow any straight device to reach the periphery of the iris. The inner end of the incision should be about 1 mm away from the limbus.

4. Inject intracameral carbachol to contract the pupil to the maximum.

5. Perform peripheral iridotomy. Slightly deepen the anterior chamber with sodium hyaluronate. Introduce a 300-μm straight Fugo blade tip through the pocket incision to reach the iris periphery. Gently press the tip and maintain it still on the iris, then very briefly activate it at medium power and high intensity. A flash may be seen and an air bubble may form. An air bubble will also form under the iris, indicating

29

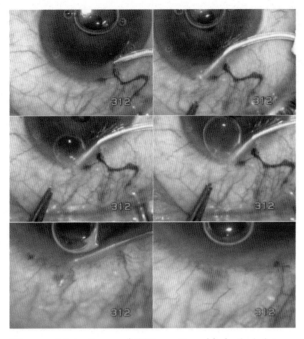

Figure 29.2. A curved 300-μm Fugo blade tip is introduced through the corneal pocket incision. It is activated and passed through the peripheral cornea into the distal subconjunctival space. The bleb made from viscous sodium hyaluronate prevents injury to the conjunctiva. The resulting track is confirmed by passing a 30-gauge (300-μm diameter) curved cannula through it.

that ablation does not extend beyond the iris. Withdraw the tip and irrigate the area to visualize the iris opening. If desired, you may perform an additional iridotomy close by (Fig. 29.2).

6. Inject more sodium hyaluronate under the limbal conjunctiva. This is needed to prevent damage to subconjunctival tissues and buttonholing by the activated tip as it exits.

7. Use a curved 300-μm Fugo blade tip to form an ab interno track. First, deepen the anterior chamber to the maximum with sodium hyaluronate. Set the Fugo blade to high power and high intensity. Carefully introduce the unactivated tip in the pocket incision and approximate it to the cornea and limbus. Keep gentle pressure on the tip in the direction of the distal subconjunctival space, then activate it momentarily. You will see a flash and feel the tip advance in the corneal tissue. A second momentary activation takes the tip into the shock-absorbing visco-elastic fluid–filled subconjunctival tissue. A sure sign of the tip emerging in the subconjunctival tissues is the appearance of cavitation bubbles beneath the conjunctiva and some sodium hyaluronate extruding through the initially made conjunctival hole at the limbus.

The track is now complete. Withdraw the curved tip in a curvilinear motion.

8. Any doubt about the formation of the track should be dispelled by introducing a curved 30-gauge cannula in the filtering track and making it appear under the conjunctiva. A 30-gauge cannula is 300 μm wide. The same cannula can be used to introduce mitomycin around the external opening.

9. Place a large air bubble in the anterior chamber. The air bubble in the anterior chamber further seals the corneal pocket incision.

10. Insert a bandage contact lens. Maintain gentle pressure on the external opening of the track to prevent shallowing of the anterior chamber.

Postoperative Management

Have the patient open the eye after 4 hours, when the effect of the facial block wears off. The bandage lens is usually in place and sits on the fluid-lifted conjunctiva. The anterior chamber is usually well formed, or it may be shallow.

Prescribe pilocarpine 2% twice a day. Even though an iridectomy is in place in line with the internal track opening, a contracted pupil ensures that the iris does not cause a block. To minimize subconjunctival fibrocytic reaction, prescribe steroid–antibiotic drops seven to eight times a day and steroid–antibiotic ointment at bedtime.

Remove the contact lens after two days. By this time, the conjunctival hole at the limbus is closed. At the end of 3 days, satisfactory anterior chamber depth and an extensive borderless bleb are usually achieved. The bleb edema reduces in a week to 10 days.

Taper steroid treatment in about 2 months.

Failure after Ab Interno Filtration

Track failure occurs for two reasons: closure of the internal opening or closure of the outer opening. Gonioscopy establishes the cause and guides the treatment.

If the internal opening is blocked with iris, pigment, or any nondescript debris, it is cleared with neodymium:yttrium–aluminum–garnet laser shots. The fluid will begin to drain and a bleb raises around the outer opening. If the inner opening is clear, the track or the outer opening needs attention.

Early raised intra-ocular pressure with nonformation of a bleb or a rapidly failing bleb may be managed by reopening the track, once again using the ab interno approach. Topical anesthesia is enough. Pressure with a curved cannula opens the original pocket incision, from where the cannula is guided into the filtration track. Fluid is injected through the cannula to clear the track and the outer opening. Depending on the situation, it may be desirable to inject antimitotic medication under the conjunctiva via the same route.

Summary

Ab interno filtration using the Fugo blade is an alternative technique for draining aqueous fluid. Further refinement of this technique is possible with improved blade tips and videovisibility through an ultrathin high-quality fiberoptic system.

Suggested Reading

Ozler SA, Hill RA, Andrew JJ, et al. Infrared laser sclerostomies. *Invest Ophthalmol Vis Sci.* 1991;32:2498.

Scimeca G. Phaco with transciliary filtration an alternative to triple procedure. *Ocular Surg News.* 2005;23:58.

Singh D, Bundela R, Agarwal A, et al. Goniotomy ab interno: "a glaucoma filtering surgery" using the Fugo plasma blade. *Ann Ophthalmol.* 2006;38:213–217.

Sugar HS. Surgical anatomy of glaucoma. *Surv Ophthalmol.* 1968;13:143.

30 Ab Externo Pretenon Filtration DALJIT SINGH and KIRANJIT SINGH

A tenon capsule is like a hornets' nest: disturb it and it strikes back. Most postsurgical complications after filtration procedures arise from the tenon capsule. The Fugo blade makes it possible to bypass the reactive tenon capsule (or at least to disturb it only minimally) while creating a basic minimum filtering track. The external pretenon approach may be transconjunctival, open, or subconjunctival.

Under a slit-lamp microscope, the normal conjunctiva close to the upper limbus looks like a delicate transparent curtain. The membrane can be moved side to side over the underlying tenon capsule with simple thumb pressure over the lid. In fact, the conjunctiva is loosely tied to the tenon capsule and is not an entirely independent layer. Free movement of the conjunctiva is facilitated by looseness of the subconjunctival tissue and especially by virtue of a small quantity of interstitial fluid. This interstitial fluid can be tremendously increased in angioneurotic edema (chemosis) or after a filtration surgery (bleb). Angioneurotic edema is diffuse; when the edema subsides, the conjunctiva completely returns to normal. A surgical bleb is a blister; it is characterized by the presence of scarlike tissue in and around it. A bleb is also subject to temporal changes such as scarring, tenon cyst formation, or ballooning and thinning. Some of these changes are a prelude to leakage, inflammation, and infection. These very changes can cause surgery failure in two ways: a rise of intra-ocular pressure or, at the other extreme, hypotony.

On the basis of our research, we believe that regulation of fluid movement beneath the conjunctiva is largely controlled by conjunctival lymphatics. They facilitate removal of excess fluid and in the process also offer some resistance.

The concept and reality of lymphatics under the conjunctiva are important for glaucoma surgery. A reliable connection between the conjunctival lymphatics and the anterior chamber without involving other tissues would solve nearly all the problems inherent in glaucoma surgery. Surgery to control glaucoma simply means the continued transfer of fluid from the anterior chamber to under the conjunctiva.

If we could pull the conjunctiva down over the limbus and create a transconjunctival filtering track through the limbus into the anterior chamber, and if that could ensure a continued track that would withstand the repairing forces of related tissues, we would need to look no further for a surgical technique for filtration. But multiple factors come into play the moment a track is made, some of which may lead to undesired results or complete failure.

Microtrack Filtration or Transconjunctival Anterior Chamber Filtration

This procedure was first performed by Daljit Singh in 2004. Conditions that warrant microtrack filtration are shown in Table 30.1. Microtrack filtration can be used in other glaucoma cases if the anterior chamber is deep. The presence of a peripheral iridectomy in the region of filtration is helpful.

Table 30.1. Conditions That Warrant Surgical Treatment with Microtrack Filtration

Angle-recession glaucoma
Traumatic hyphema
Acute and chronic uveitis with high intra-ocular pressure
Corneal ulcer with high intra-ocular pressure
Aphakic and pseudophakic glaucoma, when the anterior chamber is deep and the vitreous is restrained by the posterior capsule
Juvenile glaucoma with a deep anterior chamber

TECHNIQUE

Anesthesia

Surface anesthesia may be sufficient. To ensure that the patient feels no pain and will not move the eyeball at a critical moment during the procedure, balloon the conjunctiva with lignocaine 2% followed by 5 minutes of pressure under a pad.

Surgical Technique

1. Hold the conjunctiva lightly with a plain forceps about 3 mm from the limbus. Pull it down over the cornea to determine the amount of resistance (Figs. 30.1–30.5). When the subconjunctival connective tissue/tenon capsule is caught by the forceps, it will resist being pulled down. The less the resistance the better, because that indicates that the tenon capsule is not being dragged down.

2. Observe the limbus beneath the pulled-down conjunctiva, which should be nearly transparent. The track has to be made through the conjunctiva and the limbus without a counterpuncture. Therefore, the limbus should either be visible at all times or else physically protected from accidental touch by the Fugo blade. For better observation, stain the limbal conjunctiva with gentian violet. When the conjunctiva is pulled down, the limbus appears as a straight dark line. To avoid creating a buttonhole, do not cross this line.

3. Use a 100-μm Fugo blade tip. The tip is bent in such a way that it moves smoothly in the right direction when the track is being made. Make a dry run to ensure a smooth, practiced movement during the actual procedure.

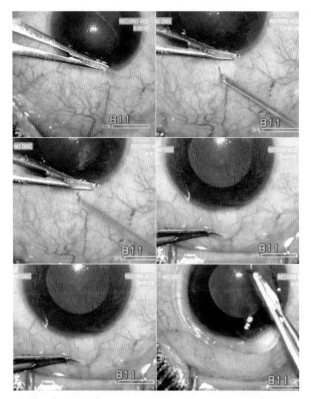

Figure 30.1. The conjunctiva is pulled over the cornea and a 100-μm Fugo blade tip is used to create a transconjunctival filtering track. A bandage lens is applied at the end of surgery.

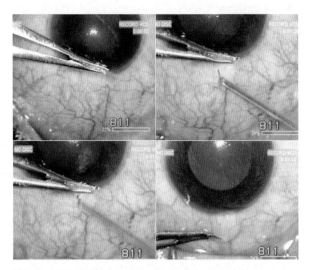

Figure 30.2. The conjunctiva is slid toward the cornea and held down at the limbus with a nonconductive crystal blund knife. A pointed 300mm Fugo blade repeatedly pushes against the sclera to enter the anterior chamber. Air is injected into the anterior chamber.

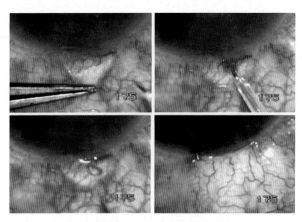

Figure 30.3. Open pretenon filtration. The detached and pulled conjunctiva reveals the insertion of tenon capsule. The filtration track is made anterior to the tenon insertion. As fluid starts draining, the conjunctiva is sutured back.

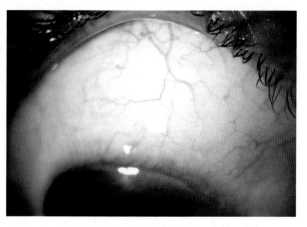

Figure 30.5. Extensive borderless bleb in a microtrack filtration that was carried out in the pretenon potential subconjunctival space.

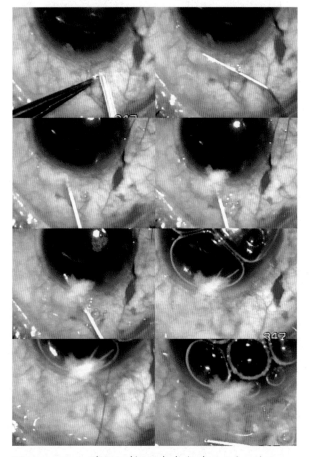

Figure 30.4. After making a hole in the conjunctiva close to the limbus, the pretenon space is opened first with saline and then ballooned with sodium hyaluronate. A 300-μm Fugo blade tip is introduced in the just-created space, turned at 45-degree angle, placed under the conjunctival insertion, activated, and pushed into the anterior chamber. Air is injected into the anterior chamber, and the initial conjunctival hole is closed with a suture.

4. The limbal area is visible through the transparent conjunctiva. It is up to the surgeon to decide at which point of the limbus to make the filtration track. Vertical entry at the posterior edge of the limbus will take the track to the anterior corneoscleral trabeculae. A track made close to the conjunctival attachment will open inside the anterior chamber far away from the corneoscleral trabeculae.

5. Either pull down the conjunctiva with a metallic forceps or slide it toward the cornea and hold it down with a noncutting nonmetallic blade (Fig. 30.1).

6. It takes only a tiny fraction of a second to make the filtration track. Keep the filament steady with very light pressure on the target tissue; it is best to hold your breath. The moment the Fugo blade is activated from the foot switch, it passes through the conjunctiva and the limbus into the anterior chamber. Fine bubbles appear in the anterior chamber from the tip. Release foot switch immediately to deactivate the Fugo blade.

7. As the ablation tip is withdrawn, aqueous ooze follows and begins to lift the conjunctiva over the external opening. You can inject air, miotics, or sodium hyaluronate (Healon) into the anterior chamber through a fine cannula. Then allow the conjunctiva to retract to its normal position. Insert a bandage contact lens to support the external opening of the track and prevent overfiltration.

In 2007, Kiranjit Singh began using the clear cornea filtration track, in which the ablating tip travels in the clear cornea before opening in the anterior chamber. The internal opening in these cases is directly visible under a slit lamp, without need of a goniolens. If internal closure of the track occurs because of an iris touch, the iris can be released by moving the iris with either a miotic or a mydriatic agent or else with a single shot of a neodymium:yttrium–aluminum–garnet (Nd:Yag) laser. In case of an iris block, my approach is to leave it alone for a couple of days while some resistance develops in the subconjunctival tissues, allowing for better control of anterior chamber depth when the iris is released. An internally blocked track can also be opened by injecting air or sodium hyaluronate through a small corneal incision.

Because of the uncertainty regarding anterior chamber depth and internal blockage with the iris after surgery, close monitoring is needed for 2 to 3 weeks, with additional minor interventions, if needed.

Surgical treatment of patients with juvenile glaucoma is particularly troublesome because of grave uncertainties connected with all surgical techniques. The conjunctiva in pediatric patients is transparent and very mobile. It is easy to make a transconjunctival track. Use a sharp, pointed Fugo blade tip to create the smallest possible internal opening right under the root of the conjunctiva. A very small internal opening and slow leakage reduces the risk of anterior chamber collapse and iris block. Place a bandage lens. Some astounding results have been obtained in young patients. The bleb formation is peculiar, in that no bleb at all appears; the conjunctiva is lifted diffusely and appears smooth and white.

Anterior chamber microfiltration cases require careful follow-up and management. The pupil needs to be contracted to keep the iris away from the internal opening of the filtration track. Cases with deep anterior chamber do better. A prefiltration laser peripheral iridotomy (PI) helps to some extent but a larger manual PI is better.

Postoperative Management

Patch the eye for 2 hours to allow the effect of the local anesthetic to wear off. Prescribe pilocarpine to be used three times a day to keep the pupil contracted, plus the usual antibiotic–steroids. Monitor the depth of the anterior chamber and the shape of the pupil. An oval pupil means iris attachment to the internal opening, which will result in deepening of the anterior chamber, followed by a rise in intra-ocular pressure.

Open Pretenon Filtration

The open technique for microtrack filtration was first performed by Dr. Hampton Roy in 2004.

Surgical Technique

1. Detach about 3 mm of the conjunctiva from the limbus.

2. Allow any bleeding point to close by itself. Do not cauterize.

3. Lift the conjunctiva to see the tenon capsule veil. The anterior limit of tenon capsule is visible. The open space anterior to it is the pretenon potential space that has been surgically opened.

4. Use a sharp, pointed 300-μm Fugo blade tip at medium power and energy to make a filtration track anterior to the visible end of the tenon capsule (Fig. 30.3). A small pointed tip produces a track that is widest (about 400 μm) outside and narrowest (about 200 μm) inside. The tip may be directed at a 45-degree angle.

5. Switch off the energy the moment cavitation bubbles appear in the anterior chamber and withdraw the tip. The fluid starts moving through the newly made track.

6. Inject intracameral carbachol to contract the pupil.

7. Inject air to deepen the anterior chamber. You may inject sodium hyaluronate in the anterior chamber to support it for a couple of hours.

8. Replace the detached conjunctiva with one or two sutures.

Closed/Subconjunctival Pretenon Filtration

It is possible to create a filtration track from the pretenon subconjunctival space to the anterior chamber using the technique described below.

Surgical Technique

1. Use a 100-μm Fugo blade tip to make a hole in the conjunctiva close to the limbus at approximately the 11 o'clock position (Fig. 30.4).

2. Balloon the conjunctive by injecting saline. Insert a 30-gauge cannula along the limbus while the saline is injected. Some fluid force plus manual force of the cannula is required to open up pretenon potential subconjunctival space.

3. Inject sodium hyaluronate through a 30-gauge cannula, starting at the distalmost part of the

30

opened subconjunctival space. This firmly raises the conjunctiva like a long blister. The blister will help protect the conjunctiva from injury during the next step.

4. Introduce a 300-μm Fugo blade tip, fully shielded right close to the tip, through the conjunctival hole and work it in for about 2 mm. Turn it toward the anterior chamber at an angle of 45 to 60 degrees. Keep the tip close to the insertion of the conjunctiva to the cornea. At this moment the sodium hyaluronate blister surrounds the tip, so the conjunctiva is not touched. Press the tip in the desired direction of movement while holding your breath, and activate the tip. In an instant, the tip crosses the cornea to enter the anterior chamber; inactivate the tip immediately. Confirm successful entry in the anterior chamber by noting the appearance of air bubbles forming inside and by visualizing the tip. Occasionally at the moment of entry, cavitation bubbles may form inside the cornea, rendering it temporarily opaque and thereby reducing visibility of the penetrating ablative tip.

5. Use a 30-gauge cannula to inject air and/or sodium hyaluronate into the anterior chamber through the newly created track.

6. Close the hole in the conjunctiva with a single suture.

Bleb formation after drainage through the pretenon potential subconjunctival space is very interesting. The fluid spreads freely under the conjunctiva and a diffuse edema is produced (Fig. 30.5).

Summary

The ab externo pretenon filtration technique can be combined with Fugo blade iridotomy or laser peripheral iridotomy. One day we may have extremely fine and stiff Fugo blade tips with electronic echo facility for interface recognition. It may then be possible to use the transconjunctival approach to selectively drain the Schlemm canal or to make minimally required anterior chamber openings that will drain aqueous fluid but do not disturb anterior chamber depth.

Suggested Readings

Sugar HS. Surgical anatomy of glaucoma. *Surv Ophthalmol.* 1968;13:143.

Ozle SA, Hill RA, Andrew JJ, et al. Infrared laser sclerostomies. *Invest Ophthalmol Vis Sci.* 1991;32:2498.

Transciliary Filtration (Singh Filtration)

C. THOMAS DOW,
KIRANJIT SINGH,
and DALJIT SINGH

"Transciliary filtration for intractable glaucoma" was first presented by Daljit Singh at the 1979 meeting of the Ophthalmological Society of the United Kingdom. In 2000, he successfully used the Fugo blade to do transciliary filtration (TCF) in a case of keratoprosthesis. Making a track through the highly vascular tissue of the ciliary body was possible because the Fugo blade ablates both tissue and blood vessels in the line of incision, and does so without the charring seen with cauterizing devices. After early successes, TCF surgery was extended to other cases of glaucoma.

TCF can be performed in any case of glaucoma in which the posterior chamber is intact and no vitreous blocks the internal opening of the filtering track. The filtration track passes through the anterior part of the sclera, the longitudinal and the circular fibers of ciliary muscle, and the ciliary processes. Since the ciliary body structure is narrowest anteriorly, the more anterior the track formation, the shorter the path to the posterior chamber.

Anatomy of the Posterior Chamber

The posterior chamber is the aqueous-filled space immediately behind the iris but in front of the lens. It is triangular in shape, the apex being toward the pupil and a 1-mm-wide base laterally. The anatomy of the lateral wall is an important consideration for TCF

procedures. The ciliary body lies posterior to the iris and has two components: the ciliary muscle and the ciliary processes. The ciliary muscle is triangular in cross section, the apex pointing posteriorly, ending at the ora serrata. The outermost longitudinal fibers attach to the corneoscleral meshwork and the scleral spur. Internal to the ciliary muscle, the ciliary processes form the pars plicata. Approximately 70 radially arrayed major ciliary processes project into the posterior chamber. Their anterior borders arise from the iris root, sweeping behind the iris to form the ciliary sulcus. These major processes are approximately 2 mm long, 0.5 mm wide, and 1 mm high and possess an irregular surface. Smaller minor ciliary processes lie between the major processes and do not project as far into the posterior chamber as the major processes. Approximately two ciliary processes exist for every millimeter of the circular ciliary body. In phakic eyes, the ciliary processes are anchored to the lens via the zonular fibers; therefore, the processes do not move freely, as the iris does. It is possible that the ciliary body as a whole moves slightly during accommodation or under the effect of mydriatics or miotics. Theoretically, this sliding movement could close a surgically created track.

During the process of TCF track formation, the ablating tip of 100 or 300 μm (the fully activated plasma tip adds an additional 100 μm) ideally enters into open space in the posterior chamber. Alternatively, it can partially or fully penetrate the ciliary body. As such, Fugo blade tip penetration into the posterior chamber can vary depending on where it successfully communicates with aqueous. When the ablating tip passes through the anterior part of the ciliary muscle, the overall distance the tip travels is less than when the track is made more posteriorly. The success of the TCF procedure depends on how the tissues of the ciliary process, ciliary muscle, sclera, and tenon capsule react to the traumatic creation of a new drainage channel and the flow of the aqueous through them.

TECHNIQUE

Anesthesia

We recommend topical anesthesia combined with peribulbar or retrobulbar injection of 1% lidocaine.

Surgical Technique

1. Open the conjunctiva at the limbus for 5 to 6 mm, then remove fibrous tissue to bare sclera (Fig. 31.1). You may extend the edge of either

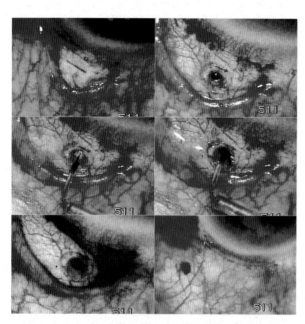

Figure 31.1. Transciliary filtration procedure. After opening the conjunctiva from the limbus a mark is made 1 mm behind the limbus. A scleral pit to the ciliary body made is with a 600-μm Fugo blade tip. The pit is beveled, especially anteriorly. An activated 100-μm Fugo blade passes through the ciliary body into the posterior chamber. Flow of aqueous is demonstrated with a drop of trypan blue. The conjunctiva is sutured at the limbus.

side of the incision radially to loosen the conjunctival flap and excise the thick tenon capsule. If you apply adjunctive mitomycin, the tenon capsule is preserved.

2. Inspect the episcleral surface. Touch any episcleral bleeding that does not stop spontaneously in 2 to 3 minutes with a 600-μm Fugo blade tip at the lowest setting. Avoid blanching the episclera with bipolar cautery to preserve normal vascularity of the scleral surface.

3. Visualize the ciliary body by transillumination, which is particularly useful in large globes. The ablation path passes through the sclera and ciliary body to the lateral wall of the posterior chamber. This is achieved with the plasma blade in two steps: first, create an ablated pit in the sclera; second, pass through the ciliary body. You must clearly understand the technique for creating the scleral pit. Make the pit with the 600-μm Fugo blade tip; it can be anywhere from 1 to 1.5 mm behind the limbus. Making a scleral pit beyond 1 mm with a 600-μm tip effectively extends the upper edge of the pit to about 1.8 to 2 mm from the limbus. The pit is vertical and extends through the suprachoroidal space. A part of the ciliary muscle may also be ablated in the process. The depth of the scleral pit occasionally makes it difficult to correctly maintain the proper plane when entering the posterior chamber. Modifications to the scleral pit can be made as follows to suit immediate surgical needs:

- The pit can be undermined in all directions to produce a larger ablated pit.

- It can be undermined anteriorly, stopping short of entering the anterior chamber. The thinned cornea can be opened later with an yttrium–aluminum–garnet (YAG) laser, if necessary. Anterior chamber filtration with TCF (Atwal's approach) can be integrated with the procedure by creating one or more tracks through the anterior wall of the scleral pit.

- It may be beveled all around, for easier egress and draining of outflowing aqueous.

It is not yet certain whether the distance of the scleral pit from the limbus has an effect on the postoperative response of the tissues. We do know that the limbus abounds in stem cells, yet we know nothing about their contribution to the success or failure of the surgery after filtration.

4. You may apply mitomycin C 0.05% (MMC) at this stage to the scleral pit, under the conjunctival flap, or both. For the former, administer MMC as a small droplet on the tip of a 30-gauge needle; dip it into the pit and leave it there for 3 to 4 minutes. For the second option, lift the conjunctival flap and apply a small sponge soaked with MMC to the episclera, being careful not to expose the edge of the flap. Vigorously irrigate the area with saline after 2 to 3 minutes.

5. To make the transciliary track, proceed with ablation through the ciliary body and its processes. The shortest distance through the ciliary body to the posterior chamber is near its attachment at the scleral spur. The depth of the ciliary body increases as the track orientation moves posteriorly. While creating an anteriorly placed track, direct the ablating tip 45 degrees. If the scleral entry point moves posteriorly, keep the 100-μm (or 300-μm) tip more parallel to the iris plane. The ideal point for scleral pit opening is as yet undetermined. Penetrating the ciliary body has many variables. You can use any of the three sizes (100, 300, or 600 μm) of Fugo blade tips.

    You may ablate the ciliary body with a 600-μm tip at medium power and medium energy, making a deep wide track completely into the posterior chamber. This is easier to do if the track is made near the anterior aspect of the suprachoroidal space.

    Stop partial ablation with a 600-μm tip at any point and create the remaining track with a 300-μm or 100-μm tip.

    Make the track through the ciliary body with the 300- or 100-μm tip (the classic TCF). Set the energy level at high and move the ablating tip slowly, thereby allowing more energy absorption and creation of a larger ablation track. Entry into the posterior chamber results in vigorous flow of aqueous with specks of pigment from the ciliary body. Occasionally, a thin stream of blood may appear that oozes for a couple of minutes. Do not try to stop it by pressure, as the blood may collect in the posterior chamber. Confirm the flow of aqueous by inserting a drop of trypan blue diluted by aqueous. Confirm the track's patency by introducing air into the scleral pit through a large-bore cannula. The air passes under the iris and through the pupil into the anterior chamber. In cases with a shallow anterior chamber with or without iris bombe the anterior chamber deepens the moment the

fluid starts begins to drain from the posterior chamber.

6. Suture the conjunctiva to the limbus.

Intra-operative Complications

Creating a scleral pit may promote bleeding, even before the ablating tip reaches the ciliary body. Avoid creating a pit at or near a large vessel. When bleeding occurs after the track has been made through the ciliary body, wait until it stops. (The site for TCF can be moved to an adjacent area.) In addition, it is advisable to irrigate the posterior chamber to make sure that no blood collects there.

A misdirected track can penetrate into the anterior chamber or into the vitreous. In the latter case, close the scleral opening with one tight suture and make a new TCF track. When the track errantly enters into the anterior chamber, direct the same ablating tip more posteriorly to and then enter the posterior chamber. Do this after filling the anterior chamber with saline and following with an air bubble; both maneuvers done to inflate the posterior chamber.

Postoperative Management

At the end of the operation, lightly patch the eye and apply a shield. Have the patient open the eye after 3 to 4 hours, when the effect of the facial block has worn off. Request that the patient instill topical steroid drops six to eight times a day. Use steroid–antibiotic ointment at bedtime.

The anterior chamber may be shallow, but is rarely, if ever, flat. Choroidal detachment is rare and recovers spontaneously. Although microscopic hyphema is frequently seen, layered hyphema is uncommon; if it does occur, it does not interfere with the filtration track. It may be left untreated and will spontaneously absorb.

The success or failure of filtration after TCF is the main postoperative concern. Early failure may occur because of a blood clot formation. Conjunctival scars may form quickly, especially in younger patients and in darkly pigmented patients. Tenon cyst formation is also a sign of a vigorous repair process. The role of the conjunctival lymphatics in the drainage of normal aqueous from the uveoscleral route and their role in aqueous management after filtration surgery should not be underestimated. Every effort should be made to minimize trauma: mechanical, thermal, or chemical. Histologic studies of TCF-operated animal or cadaver eyes are not yet available.

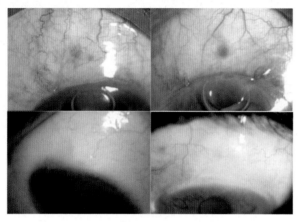

Figure 31.2. Top: Blebs in the early postoperative period. **Bottom:** The same TCF blebs years after surgery.

Blebs after Transciliary Filtration

Although nothing is standard about blebs in any particular glaucoma surgery technique, TCF blebs have certain characteristics. Because the TCF track is direct, it promotes symmetric aqueous distribution under the conjunctiva and produces a broad, borderless bleb (Fig. 31.2).

Concurrent Transciliary Filtration and Phaco-emulsification

Because of predictable adequate anterior chamber depth, TCF may be considered a preferable filtering procedure to combine with phaco-emulsification. Scleral ablation is done before phaco-emulsification, whereas penetration into the posterior chamber is completed after phaco-emulsification. It is important to pay attention to adequate volume reconstitution of the anterior and posterior chambers at the end of the phaco procedure to ensure ample egress of aqueous fluid when the posterior chamber is entered.

Neovascular Glaucoma

Cases of neovascular glaucoma are treated well by TCF because this procedure requires no manipulation of the iris. Oozing blood from the angle resulting from operative relative hypotony usually does not interfere with the aqueous outflow through the posterior chamber. We suggest the concurrent use of intravitreal bevacizumab (off-label).

Reoperation after Transciliary Filtration

The two approaches to reoperation after TCF are (1) opening the conjunctiva from the limbus and revising the track (open revision) and (2) performing transconjunctival transciliary filtration (TCTCF) (closed revision).

Open Revision of Transciliary Filtration

Surgical Technique

Open the conjunctiva as previously described. If present, scar or tenon cyst formation is removed from the field with the 600-μm Fugo blade tip. The filtration track may start working spontaneously or may be revived by additional ablative treatment in the same site. Loss of filtration may occur because of a clot within the pit or deeper in the track. Once retreated, verify the egress of the fluid with a drop of trypan blue and resuture the conjunctiva (Fig. 31.3)

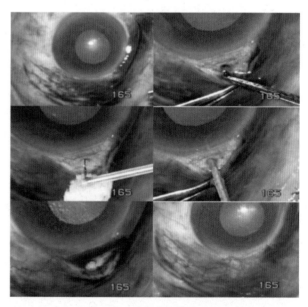

Figure 31.3. Filtration after failed TCF. Lymphatic charting showed a healthy network. On opening the conjunctiva, a blood clot was observed in the scleral pit. The track was reopened with a 100-μm Fugo blade tip, aqueous flow was confirmed with trypan blue, and the conjunctiva was sutured back to the limbus.

31

Closed Revision of Transciliary Filtration

Surgical Technique

In closed revision of TCF (TCTCF) (Fig. 31.4), pull down and stretch redundant conjunctiva while passing an activated 300-μm Fugo blade tip through the conjunctiva into the old TCF track until it draws aqueous from the posterior chamber. The relative ease and efficacy of TCTCF surgery have led some to consider TCTCF as a primary surgery for glaucoma.

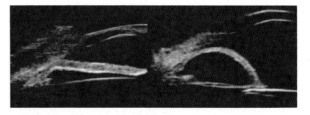

Figure 31.5. Ultrasound biomicroscopy aids in visualizing the posterior chamber, finding the best site for filtration and enabling the surgeon to determine the best anatomic approach to the posterior chamber.

Role of Ultrasound Biomicroscopy in Transciliary Filtration

Ultrasound biomicroscopy (UMB) allows visualization of the anatomy of the posterior chamber (Fig. 31.5). UMB images orient the surgeon to the site of the scleral pit and the direction of the ciliary body ablating tip. It is possible to judge the volume of the posterior chamber and the expected flow of the aqueous when the posterior chamber is reached.

Future Role of Fiberoptic Cameras

Currently, the operating microscope provides lighting and magnification of the operative field. Ablating the ciliary body is done blindly, assisted primarily by the surgeon's instinct and sense of direction. Microfiberoptic cameras with amazing resolution are expected to become available in the future. These cameras are capable of revealing the internal as well as the external microanatomic detail of the surgical site, allowing for complete control of Fugo blade ablation. This technologic advance will bring about a new era of directly visualized microsurgery that will likely become the standard for glaucoma surgery.

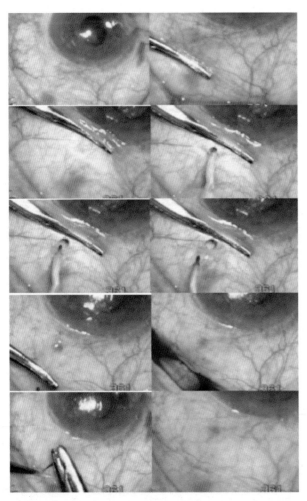

Figure 31.4. Revision of a filtering bleb. The conjunctiva from the fornix side is folded over the original track. A 300-μm Fugo blade tip ablates through the conjunctiva and the previously created track, and aqueous begins to flow. The conjunctival opening is closed with a suture. A broad, low bleb is the result.

Summary

After a century-long search for better anterior chamber filtration, posterior chamber filtration is an interesting alternative. It is accomplished without disturbing the existing natural drainage and, in fact, enhances functioning by reducing the potential for iris bombe and encroachment on the corneoscleral trabeculae.

Creating a filtration path through the ciliary body was not practical prior to the development of the Fugo plasma blade. The idea of TCF reemerged because of the Fugo blade's unique cutting and ablating capabilities. The lightweight, small, battery-operated Fugo blade unit facilitates TCF procedures in even the most remote corners of the world.

Suggested Readings

Dow CT, deVenecia G. Transciliary filtration (Singh procedure) with the Fugo plasma blade. *Ann Ophthalmol (Skokie)*. 2008 Spring;40(1):8–14.

Fugo R. Regarding transciliary filtration. *Trop Ophthalmol*. 2002;2:7–8.

Fugo R. Transciliary filtration procedure offers new approach to glaucoma. *Ocular Surgery News*. 2005; 23:4–26.

Guttman C. Transciliary filtration provides improved safety and simplicity. *Ophthalmol Times*. 2005;30:28.

Kent C. FDA approves new glaucoma filtration procedure. *Rev Ophthalmol*. 2004;11:6–8.

Kent C. Transciliary filtration—without bleeding. *Ophthalmol Manage*. 2002;6:84–87.

Singh D. Singh micro-filtration for glaucoma: a new technique. *Trop Ophthalmol*. 2001;1:7–11.

Singh D. Transciliary filtration & lymphatics of conjunctiva—a tale of discovery. *Trop Ophthalmol*. 2002;2:9–13.

Singh D, Singh K. Transciliary filtration using the Fugo blade. *Ann Ophthalmol*. 2002;34:183–187.

Tenon Cyst DALJIT SINGH and KIRANJIT SINGH

32

The proliferative fibrotic response of the tenon capsule leads to filtration failure. Keloid formation or "sclerification" of the subconjunctival connective tissue/tenon capsule can happen slowly over weeks or months, or it may take effect within days. The filtering bleb progressively shrinks and intra-ocular pressure increases. Forcing the fluid out of the eye with massage and pressure produces progressively less result and eventually fails. The tenon cyst has a characteristic clinical appearance: elevated localized bleb, prominent surface vessels, and patent internal opening on gonioscopy. Intervention with a needle or injection of fluorouracil or mitomycin C are ways to salvage the failing blebs. But the only recourse is to excise the tenon cyst.

The cause of bleb encapsulation is not known. Male sex, topical corticosteroids, previous argon laser trabeculoplasty, and use of beta-blockers are some potential risk factors for the development of an encapsulated filtering bleb. Glaucoma valves also fail by encapsulation. The incidence of bleb encapsulation has been reported to be anywhere from 3 to 30% in trabeculectomy cases.

The conjunctiva over the cyst is generally, but not always, mobile. Its outer edge may adhere to the conjunctiva, requiring patience when cutting and reflecting the tissue. The cyst may be exposed by making a fornix-based or a limbal-based conjunctival flap. Sclerification and the edge of the tenon cyst extend much further than its apparent size.

Although optimal management of bleb encapsulation has not been defined, we have used the Fugo blade to address tenon cysts as discussed below.

Transconjunctival Restoration of Filtration

We use this approach when it appears that the cyst wall is thin and does not extend beyond the filtration area, the conjunctiva is mobile over it, and tissues appear normal—not inflamed or irritated.

Surgical Technique

1. Check the motility of the conjunctiva over the cyst using a plain forceps. Make a mark using gentian violet on the conjunctiva near the proximal edge. When you pull the conjunctiva down, this spot marks the limit that should not be crossed in order to prevent buttonholing.

2. Direct and gently press an inactivated 100-μm Fugo blade tip at the intended entry point. Press the foot paddle momentarily, which activates the tip and takes it through the cyst wall. Another indicator of successful breach of the cyst is the entry of cavitation bubbles into the anterior chamber. The outflowing aqueous raises the conjunctiva as a large bleb, and the anterior chamber becomes shallow.

3. Use a diamond knife to make a side port incision through which to inject sodium hyaluronate to deepen the anterior chamber. Now the anterior chamber is not leaking, and a large conjunctival bleb now exists, with a hole that was made along with the transconjunctival track. At this stage it is

32

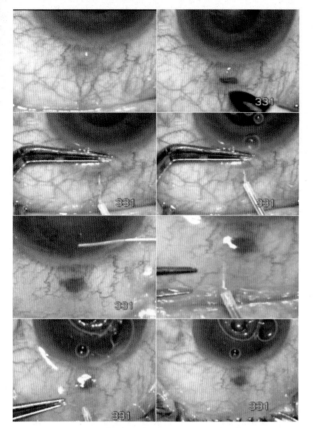

Figure 32.1. A small tenon cyst developed after microtrack filtration. A mark is made with gentian violet to prevent counterpuncture when the mobile conjunctiva is displaced downward and the cyst is opened transconjunctivally with a 100-μm Fugo blade tip. The conjunctiva is ballooned up with the outflowing aqueous. The anterior chamber is deepened with sodium hyaluronate through a 0.75-mm corneal pocket incision. One or more additional openings are made in the tenon cyst through the conjunctival opening.

easy to pass the ablation tip through the hole, enter under the conjunctiva, and make additional openings in the cyst.

4. The conjunctival hole may or may not be sutured (Fig. 32.1).

Cyst Removal after Reflecting the Conjunctiva

This approach can be used to manage large cysts with thick walls. The conjunctival flap may be fornix-based or limbus-based. Dissection is not easy if the cyst is firmly adhered to the conjunctiva. In such cases, part or all of the conjunctiva over the cyst must

be sacrificed. When the cyst is fully exposed, it is found to be much wider than it appeared before surgery.

Surgical Technique

1. Use a 300- or 600-μm Fugo tip at medium power setting to ablate the cyst, starting from the periphery and progressing toward the center. When the cyst wall is breached, the aqueous flows outward and the eye becomes soft.
2. Remove the last portion of the cyst wall, or it may be left as a partial cover for the filtration track.
3. Suture the conjunctiva (Fig. 32.2).

In a fornix-based approach, greater risk of losing the conjunctiva over the cyst exists. In a limbus-based approach, dissection is done from underneath, and the anterior wall of the cyst may be left alone or merely thinned, but not breached, thereby preserving the conjunctiva over it. However, one clumsy move or an attempt to ablate a little more will create a buttonhole, which then necessitates suturing both at the limbus and toward the fornix.

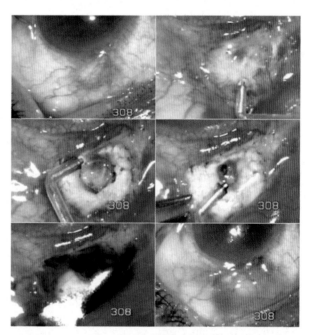

Figure 32.2. A case of transciliary filtration. The cyst is apparently small but turns out to be much bigger when it is exposed. All of the cyst wall is ablated using a 600-μm Fugo blade tip, leaving a small loose leaking cap (as seen by the flow of trypan blue) over the filtering track. The conjunctiva is pulled down and sutured to the limbus.

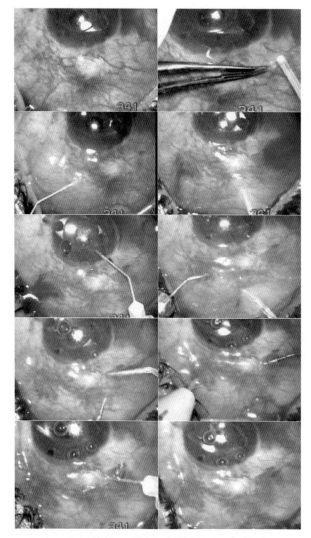

Subconjunctival Approach for Subtotal Tenon Cyst Ablation

The subtotal destruction of the tenon cyst wall and its base is relatively less traumatic than the open approach. No hemorrhaging occurs, and ablation debris is washed away with copious irrigation under the conjunctiva. We have tried to use a vitrector to ablate tenon capsule; two ports were made in the conjunctiva, one for irrigation and the other for the vitrectomy/tenonectomy tip. But only very thin-walled cysts could be managed partially, and a high risk of bleeding and conjunctival buttonholing existed.

A special Fugo blade tip is used for the subconjunctival approach. The tip has a 300-μm filament surrounded by a thick sleeve of nonstick material, so that the tip is naked for about 0.125 mm on the front and about 0.25 mm on the underside. When the tip is moved in the process of ablation, it will not threaten overlying conjunctiva.

Surgical Technique

1. Make a conjunctival hole with a plasma blade with a 100-μm tip, near the limbus about 3 mm from the edge of the cyst (Fig. 32.3).

2. Balloon the conjunctiva around the cyst with saline, followed by visco-elastic material. Injecting the visco-elastic material stretches the conjunctival hole.

3. Insert the tenon ablation tip under the conjunctiva until it reaches the edge of the cyst.

4. Use medium power and medium energy for ablation. First, ablate the nearest wall, releasing the blocked aqueous and further raising the conjunctival bleb. Make a stab incision in the anterior chamber and inject visco-elastic material to halt further aqueous flow under the conjunctiva. Reintroduce the ablation tip and move it from the limbal side upward to open up the tenon cyst as much as possible. In this process, the side walls and the scleral side of the cyst are destroyed, while the anterior wall and the conjunctiva over it are saved from ablation. If necessary, inject more visco-elastic material under the conjunctiva, so that the ablation tip poses no threat of counterpuncture.

5. Depending on the situation, you may approach the tenon cyst from one or two additional conjunctival openings: one from the opposite side and one from above. You may inject the area of the cyst with 0.04% mitomycin for 4 to 5 minutes and then rinse it copiously with saline. Its entry into the anterior chamber is blocked by the sodium hyaluronate inside the chamber.

6. Close the conjunctival holes with sutures, or you may leave them alone to close naturally (Fig. 32.4).

Figure 32.3. Three conjunctival holes are made with a 100-μm Fugo blade tip, and the conjunctiva is raised with saline and sodium hyaluronate. The cyst is first breached with an ablation tip introduced through the upper opening. The anterior chamber is filled with sodium hyaluronate, injected through a stab incision. The ablation process is carried out through all the three conjunctiva, while the conjunctiva is kept raised by continued irrigation under it. The process is considered complete when a cannula introduced from the side can be moved freely up and down. Mitomycin 0.04% was irrigated under the cyst and rinsed by irrigation after 4 minutes.

32

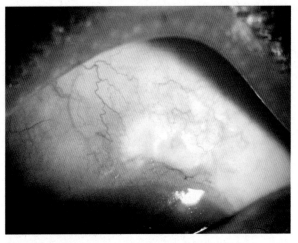

Figure 32.4. The same patient as in Figure 32.3, 2 months after surgery.

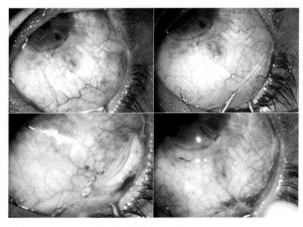

Figure 32.5. A failed glaucoma valve due to tenon cyst. Incision in the conjunctiva is followed by excision of a strip of the tenon cyst that also exposes the edge of the valve. The conjunctiva is closed with sutures.

Tenon Cyst over the Glaucoma Valve

A frequent cause of glaucoma valve failure is the formation of a thick tenon cyst over it, but these cysts are easy to manage. Make a bold 100-μm tip incision over the valve, going through the conjunctiva and the cyst wall. The cyst wall usually does not adhere to the conjunctiva or to the valve. Excise a strip of the cyst wall, including the part over the edge of the valve, with the same Fugo blade tip, exposing the valve; the restrained aqueous flows out from under the edge of the valve. Nothing more needs to be done. Suture the conjunctiva (Fig. 32.5).

Summary

The Fugo blade is a useful tool to manage all cases of tenon cysts. The size and thickness of the cyst wall are immaterial. Either an open or a closed approach can be used. Bloodless, nondissective destruction/ablation of the tenon cyst through tiny holes in the conjunctiva guarantees quick recovery. Injection of antimitotic agents or application of pressure to the eyeball to squeeze out the aqueous fluid is not needed.

Suggested Reading

Gutiérrez-Díaz E, Montero-Rodríguez M, Julve San Martín A, et al. [Incidence of encapsulated bleb after filtering surgery.] [Article in Spanish.] *Arch Soc Esp Oftalmol.* 2001; 76:279–284.

Cyclodialysis DALJIT SINGH

33

I n traditional cyclodialysis, an incision is made in the sclera some distance from the limbus to reach the suprachoroidal space. Through this scleral slit, an instrument introduced into the suprachoroidal space enters the anterior chamber after breaking the scleral spur. The scleral spur is broken for about 2 mm on either side of the entry point. The ciliary body detaches from the sclera, and a cleft is created that allows the fluid to freely enter the suprachoroidal space. From there the aqueous is supposed to flow through the sclera to the subconjunctival space. Cyclodialysis using the Fugo blade follows along the same lines, but in a different and more effective manner, as described below.

CASE STUDY

Case 1: Buphthalmos

The patient was 5-year-old suffering from buphthalmos. The eye had suffered trauma and had become a painful blind eye. There was no light perception in the affected eye. The child had been in severe pain for over a month and was getting no relief from medication. The parents were desperate to end the child's suffering, even if that meant that the eye had to be removed.

The eye was hard. There was blood in the anterior chamber, and a streak of blood lined the back of the cornea at the site of a huge tear in the Descemet membrane. We performed surgery as described below.

Surgical Technique

1. Use a 100-μm Fugo blade tip to make a hole in the conjunctiva close to its attachment to the cornea. Balloon the conjunctiva with lignocaine injected with a cannula through the hole.

2. Make a large conjunctival incision close to its corneal attachment, again using a Fugo blade (Fig. 33.1). In our case, there was no bleeding.

3. Retract the conjunctiva upward (fornix-based) for almost 7 to 8 mm.

4. Roughly judge the location of the angle of the anterior chamber by visual inspection; you can also judge it by transillumination with fiber light. In our case, we needed to incise the sclera 4 to 5 mm posterior to the chamber angle.

5. Use a 500-μm Fugo blade at low power and energy settings to make an approximately 1.5-mm-long gutter on the sclera parallel to the limbus. Deepen the gutter slowly until the ciliary body is visible. Carefully ablate any remnant of sclera to provide a sharp and clear edge.

6. Introduce a long, thin cannula under the anterior edge of the scleral gutter. Advance the cannula gradually, hugging the sclera, until it reaches and then breaks the scleral spur. Extend the spur break for about 2 mm on either side. In our case, some blood-stained aqueous issued from the scleral gutter.

7. Inject air into the anterior chamber through the same route.

8. Make a 500-μm hole in the wide limbus.

9. Trypan blue dropped on the scleral gutter and the anteriorly placed hole is rinsed away by the draining aqueous.

10. Suture the conjunctiva back to the cornea.

Figure 33.2 shows functioning cyclodialysis after the procedure.

33

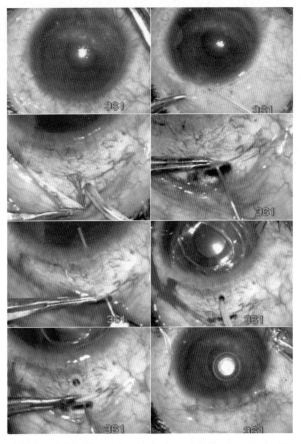

Figure 33.1. The ballooned conjunctiva is incised with Fugo blade. A 500-μm Fugo blade tip is used to make a scleral gutter. Cyclodialysis is done with a long 30-gauge cannula. A 500-μm track is made at the limbus, over the cyclodialysis track. A cannula passed under the sclera appears at the limbal hole before passing into the anterior chamber. The conjunctival flap is sutured back.

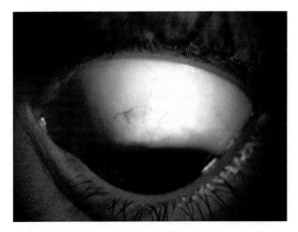

Figure 33.2. Functioning cyclodialysis in a case of buphthalmos (Case 1).

Case 2: Deformed Anterior Segment

If the cyclodialysis cleft and the scleral gutter remain open, a filtration track will begin functioning. To facilitate aqueous flow, a 300-μm Fugo blade tip can be used to ablate a subscleral groove by moving the activated tip from the edge of the scleral gutter into the anterior chamber. The activated tip is directed anteriorly toward the sclera as it moves toward the anterior chamber. Entry into the anterior chamber is confirmed by the appearance of cavitation bubbles within the chamber. We treated a 65-year-old patient with pseudophakia who had a deformed anterior segment from earlier antiglaucoma operations. The patient suffered bouts of pain and had a high intraocular pressure. The steps of the operation are given below.

TECHNIQUE

Anesthesia

Administer facial and retrobulbar block.

Surgical Technique

1. After making a bloodless puncture with a 100-μm Fugo blade tip, balloon the conjunctiva with saline. Make an 8-mm-long incision in the conjunctiva with the same tool, as close to the limbus as possible.

2. Retract the conjunctiva to expose the sclera (Fig. 33.3).

3. Use a 500-μm Fugo blade tip to make a scleral gutter approximately 1.5 mm long to reach the ciliary body. Perform ablation at medium power and a high energy setting.

4. Because the scleral pit has steep walls, bevel the upper edge of the scleral pit to facilitate the next step.

5. Insert a cyclodialysis spatula under the anterior edge of the scleral gutter and traverse the suprachoroidal space, breaking the scleral spur and entering the anterior chamber. Do not break the scleral spur on either side, as is usually done. When the spatula is withdrawn, the aqueous fluid does not flow out, so the scleral pit remains dry.

7. A drop of trypan blue over the scleral pit is washed away by the draining aqueous.

8. Suture the conjunctiva.

This technique can be used to introduce a seton or glaucoma valve tubing in the suprachoroidal space.

This procedure does not resemble classical cyclodialysis. Instead, a filtering track has been made between the anterior chamber and a gap in the sclera at the site of the gutter. Aqueous fluid can reach the suprachoroidal space through the hole created by the Fugo blade in the angle of the anterior chamber. It can spread out or pass out of the scleral gutter.

Insertion of the cyclodialysis spatula and, especially, the 300-μm Fugo blade tip are greatly facilitated by first beveling the superior edge of the gutter.

The scleral gutter approach has been used to drain both dark suprachoroidal hemorrhage and pale yellow suprachoroidal fluid in cases of choroidal detachment.

Summary

Cyclodialysis was introduced by Heine in 1905.[1] It was performed as an alternative to filtering surgery, especially in aphakic eyes, or in combination with cataract surgery. Use of the technique has largely been abandoned, however, owing to its unpredictable results, a lack of improvements to the technique over the years, and the development of better procedures. Use of the Fugo blade, however, has revived the surgeon's ability to use the suprachoroidal space as a conduit for aqueous fluid in selected cases.

Reference

1. Schaffer RN, Weiss DL. Concerning cyclodialysis and hypotony. *Arch Ophthalmol*. 1962;68:25–31.

Suggested Reading

Alpar JJ. Sodium hyaluronate (Healon) in cyclodialysis. *CLAO J*. 1985;11:201–204.

Roy FH. *Master techniques in ophthalmic surgery*. Philadelphia, Pa: Williams & Wilkins, 1995.

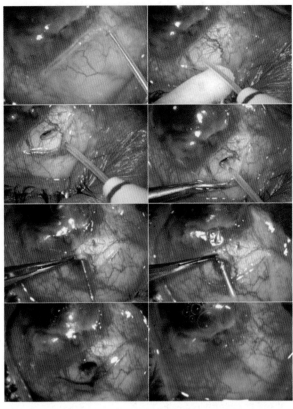

Figure 33.3. The conjunctiva is incised with a 100-μm Fugo blade tip. The scleral gutter is created and the upper edge of the scleral pit is beveled using a 500-μm tip. A cyclodialysis spatula separates the sclera from the ciliary body and enters the anterior chamber. The 300-μm tip of Fugo blade follows the same track, but also ablates the undersurface of the sclera. The fluid flows out as the tip is withdrawn. Trypan blue dye gets washed away. The conjunctiva is sutured back.

6. Make a gutter with a 300-μm Fugo blade tip on the underside of the sclera from the scleral pit to the anterior chamber. Ablate the anterior edge of the scleral gutter and advance the tip toward the anterior chamber, pressing it toward the sclera at all times to create a channel underneath it. Once the anterior chamber is reached, withdraw the ablating tip. The aqueous starts flowing from the anterior chamber to the scleral pit.

34 Neovascular Glaucoma

DALJIT SINGH, KIRANJIT SINGH, and C. THOMAS DOW

The story of neovascular glaucoma never ends. The treatment—both medical and surgical—is difficult and failures are common. Lifelong follow-up and appropriate management are required. The Fugo blade, with its unique cutting properties, now offers a better way to handle this intractable condition.

The most important causes of neovascular glaucoma are central retinal vein occlusion, proliferative diabetic retinopathy, and branch-vein occlusion. Vascular endothelial growth factor is considered to be the cause of new vessel formation. Rubeosis of the iris and growth of a fibrovascular membrane over the trabecular meshwork cause a rise in intra-ocular pressure. Delayed diagnosis and unsuccessful medical management of neovascular glaucoma are common, as is the relentless progression of the disease toward painful glaucoma and blindness.

Surgical methods currently used to treat neovascular glaucoma include trabeculectomy with or without an antifibrotic agent, valve-implant surgery, and cyclodestructive procedures. Filtration surgery for neovascular glaucoma is particularly challenging. The fragile blood vessels from the angle of the anterior chamber start leaking the moment intra-ocular pressure falls during the course of any filtration surgery.

Dr. Singh first used the Fugo blade to treat neovascular glaucoma in a patient with an extremely painful blind eye. The patient's intra-ocular pressure was over 60 mm Hg. After giving the patient a retrobulbar injection of lignocaine, Singh and Dow made a single transconjunctival transciliary filtration (TCF) track with a 100-μm Fugo blade tip. The patient never suffered pain in that eye again, although his intra-ocular pressure remained at around 35 mm Hg while taking local antiglaucoma medication.

We became interested in TCF for neovascular glaucoma for several reasons:

1. No trauma to the vascularized angle of the anterior chamber occurs. The iris with rubeosis is not traumatized by iridectomy.

2. A filtration channel is created through the ciliary body, which is free from neovascularization. No fibrovascular membrane forms at the site of the inner opening behind the iris. The filtration track is made through the relatively healthy tissues.

3. Leaked blood in the anterior chamber does not conflict with the filtration track and is less of a cause of surgical failure than other more important factors, like fibrosis and inflammation.

We have operated on over a dozen cases of neovascular glaucoma, using two techniques: TCF after making a fornix-based conjunctival flap and the direct transconjunctival approach. In nearly half the cases, blood oozed from the angle of the anterior chamber during the course of surgery. Postoperative hyphema did not drain through the TCF track, but absorbed spontaneously over a period of days or weeks. Filtration failed as a result of subconjunctival scarring or tenon cyst formation. Reoperation was done whenever there was failure (almost 50% of cases). None of the patients who had progressed to a painful blind eye needed relief through a retrobulbar alcohol injection, a cyclodestructive procedure, or enucleation.

Postoperative follow-up is particularly tricky because most of these patients are occupied with more pressing diabetic, cardiac, and renal conditions.

In all operated cases, neovascularization of the iris was seen to regress or disappear as long as the intra-ocular pressure was not high. The vision of these six patients was preserved; they all had branch-vein occlusion.

The ups and downs of surgical care of neovascular glaucoma are illustrated by the description of one patient, as shown below.

CASE STUDIES

Case 1

A 55-year-old woman with diabetes and multiple systemic problems had lost the vision in one eye to retinal detachment; the intra-ocular pressure in the other eye was over 40 mm Hg. There were vascular changes in the iris and the angle. Medical management with multiple local drops and oral acetazolamide (Diamox) were successful for about 6 months, after which the pressure shot up to 50 mm Hg and her vision rapidly deteriorated. Surgery was decided on.

As a preliminary treatment, paracentesis was done and bevacizumab (Avastin) injected in the anterior chamber. The operation was done the next day as described below.

Surgical Technique

1. Visualize the surgical limbus under the conjunctiva. Make a depression mark 1 mm behind the limbus by pressing on it with the noncutting back side of a diamond blade (Fig. 34.1).

2. Slide the loose conjunctiva about 4 to 5 mm proximal to the depression mark over the underlying tenon capsule, using the edge of a nonmagnetic noncutting blade. In our case, we used a purposely blunted diamond knife. In this state it did not cut when pressed on the eyeball, but it did hold down the dragged conjunctiva in the gutter made moments before. The gutter was about 1 mm away from the limbus.

3. Set a 300-μm Fugo blade tip at medium power and high intensity. The tip is bent at a convenient angle to easily direct it toward the posterior chamber. Lightly push the activated tip along the edge of the diamond conjunctival rectractor. It instantly goes through the conjunctiva and partly through the sclera. Withdraw the tip, and touch it

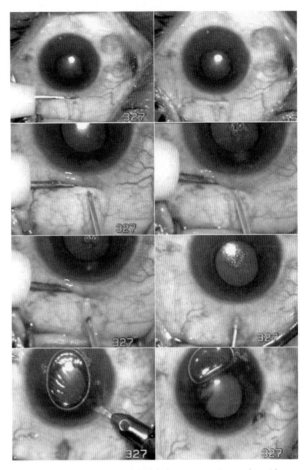

Figure 34.1. A linear scleral depression is made with a blunt nonmagnetic device. The conjunctiva is slid toward the limbus, activated, and pressed into the depression. Transconjunctival transciliary filtration is done with a 300-μm Fugo blade. Irrigation and air injection is done through the transciliary track. Sodium hyaluronate (Healon) is injected through a stab incision.

very briefly deeper in the track another two to three times until fluid starts to flow from the posterior chamber. Small air bubbles issue from behind the iris as they enter the anterior chamber. This ensures that the track is indeed in the posterior chamber.

4. In our case, blood was seen leaking from many points in the angle of the anterior chamber. We therefore irrigated the eye from the TCF track. It helped to some extent, yet the leakage continued. To stem, it a large air bubble was introduced through the posterior chamber track (Fig. 34.2).

5. For a further tamponade, make a stab incision at the limbus and inject sodium hyaluronate (Healon) into the anterior chamber.

34

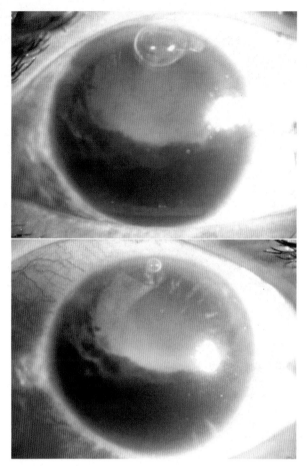

Figure 34.2. The anterior chamber before and 1 day after sodium hyaluronate removal.

It is not certain whether the injection of sodium hyaluronate helped in our case to retard the blood leaking from the fragile vessels in the angle, but it did raise the intra-ocular pressure. It may have do so by pressing the iris backward, which caused the internal opening in the ciliary body to close, and by occluding the angle of the anterior chamber. Therefore, as an emergency, sodium hyaluronate was aspirated within 4 hours of surgery. The blood ooze seen in the anterior chamber at the time of surgery was now manifesting as a blackball hemorrhage occupying the lower half of the anterior chamber (Fig. 34.2). It was left alone for the time being.

Postoperative Management

There was no significant spontaneous blood clearing in the coming days and the patient felt her vision slipping away. On the 4th postoperative day, urokinase (10,000 units per milliliter) was repeatedly irrigated in

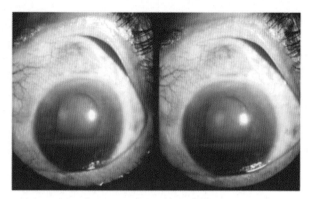

Figure 34.3. The anterior chamber 3 days after urokinase wash. The dark blood is clearly visible. The bleb is still functional.

the anterior chamber to attack the blackball hemorrhage. There was partial success. The irrigating process pushed some dissolved blood through the transciliary track under the conjunctiva that appeared as a blood stain at the outer opening (Fig. 34.3). Intra-ocular pressure was still under control.

The patient was comfortable and the blood was allowed to absorb spontaneously; eventually no blood remained. Intra-ocular pressure rose once again but was controlled with local and oral medications. Finally, 2 months later, the surgery failed completely. The patient was not in pain, but her sight was in jeopardy. A reoperation was done in an adjoining area, exactly as performed in the first procedure. Transconjunctival TCF was performed in an adjoining healthy area (Fig. 34.4). One month after the surgery (Figs. 34.5 and 35.6), the patient's intra-ocular pressure had returned to normal and the anterior chamber was clear.

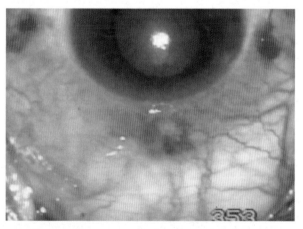

Figure 34.4. Transconjunctival transciliary filtration has been repeated on the temporal side of the failed track.

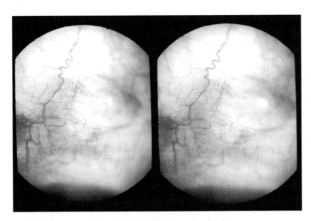

Figure 34.5. The filtering bleb under high power 1 month after repeat surgery. The image shows very clearly that the bleb is widespread and the conjunctiva is healthy and transparent.

Surgical Technique

1. After detaching the conjunctiva from the limbus and obtaining hemostasis, make a scleral pit on the sclera 1.5 mm from the limbus (Fig. 34.7).
2. Apply a small sponge soaked with mitomycin to the undersurface of the retracted conjunctiva.
3. Clear blood from the anterior chamber by irrigation and aspiration through two different ports.
4. Reach the posterior chamber by ablating through the ciliary body with a 100-μm Fugo blade at maximum energy settings.
5. Repeat two-port irrigation and aspiration to wash out the anterior chamber.
6. Suture the conjunctiva.
7. Inject intravitreal bevacizumab.

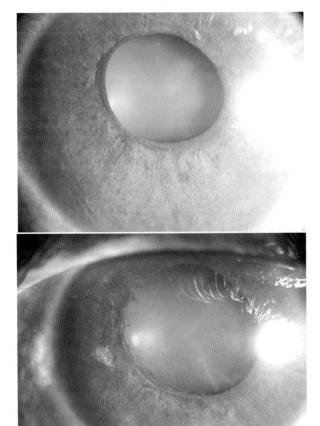

Figure 34.6. Preoperatively there was new vessel formation close to the pupil. One month after surgery, no neovascularization is apparent.

Case 2

The following case describes TCF surgery in a case of neovascular glaucoma. The anterior chamber was full of blood.

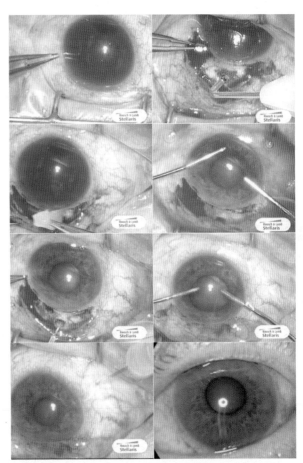

Figure 34.7. Top left to bottom right: Neovascular glaucoma with hyphema; transciliary filtration scleral ablation; mitomycin application; anterior chamber washout of hyphema; transciliary filtration penetration; repeat anterior chamber washout after wound suture; intravitreal bevacizumab injected; patient's appearance on 6th postoperative day shows complete regression of rubeosis (intra-ocular pressure, 7 mm Hg).

Summary

Neovascular glaucoma is an intractable disease, and surgery often fails. The Fugo blade offers the surgeon a variety of credible solutions for the treatment of this condition. Transconjunctival TCF seems to be the least traumatic choice and can be redone at the original failed track or in an adjoining area.

New vessel formation in the iris decreases or disappears as the intra-ocular pressure is controlled. The use of anti–vascular endothelial growth factor medicine in the anterior chamber probably helps. We have limited experience, but mitomycin might be a useful adjunct to treatment. Dark-skinned patients do not have a predictable response.

Suggested Reading

Albert DM, Jakobiec FA. Neovascular glaucoma. In: *Principles and practice of ophthalmology, clinical ophthalmology* [book on CD-ROM]. Philadelphia, Pa: Saunders, chapter 215.

Epstein DL, Allingham RR, Schuman JS. *Chandler and Grant's glaucoma*. 4th ed. Philadelphia, Pa: Lea & Febiger, 1997:309–318.

Gupta V, Agarwal HC. Contact trans-scleral diode laser cyclophotocoagulation treatment for refractory glaucomas in the Indian population. *Indian J Ophthalmol.* 2000; 48:295–300.

Lieberman MF, Ewing RH. Drainage implant surgery for refractory glaucoma. *Int Ophthalmol Clin.* 1990;30:198–208.

Parodi MB, Iacono P. Photodynamic therapy with verteporfin for anterior segment neovascularizations in neovascular glaucoma. *Am J Ophthalmol.* 2004;138:157–158.

Shields MB. *Textbook of glaucoma*. 4th ed. 1998:269–286.

Sivak-Callcott JA, O'Day DM, Gass JD. Evidence-based recommendations for the diagnosis and treatment of neovascular glaucoma. *Ophthalmology.* 2001;108:1767–1800.

Part G
The Anterior Segment

Anterior Vitrectomy DALJIT SINGH

Vitrectomy is mandatory when the vitreous presents in the anterior chamber during the course of cataract surgery. It is also done when a planned posterior capsulorrhexis is performed in pediatric patients. A manual vitrector does this job superbly, combining saline irrigation and vitrectomy simultaneously. Irrigation from the same port increases the amount of vitrectomy needed, so irrigation from a second port is preferred. The end point of vitrectomy is a matter of judgment. Most often the vitreous is cut much more than initially planned.

My colleagues and I have used the Fugo blade to perform a small anterior vitrectomy with great ease, as illustrated in the following example.

CASE STUDY

Case: Congenital Fibrovascular Cataract

The 2-year-old had a congenital fibrovascular cataract. The central dense fibrovascular mass was invaded by many blood vessels from the ciliary body. The surgery was done as described below.

Surgical Technique

1. Fix an iris claw intraocular lens in place.

2. Keep the anterior chamber deep by injecting methylcellulose from the side port, and gently insert the Fugo blade under the intraocular lens. Ablate the periphery of the cataract along with invading blood vessels with plasma energy. In our case, during this process, a large hyaloid vessel was revealed. We cut this vessel too by carrying the ablating tip behind the fibrovascular mass into the vitreous (Fig. 35.1).

3. When the fibrovascular mass is freed from all sides, pull it out through the incision. In our case, many vitreous strands were attached to the mass as it was brought out. We cut the strands with the Fugo blade outside the incision line.

4. We saw vitreous strands coming out from under the upper edge of the intraocular lens and sticking to the iris and the incision line.

5. To visualize the vitreous in the anterior chamber, the particulate form of steroid, dilute triamcinolone was used to irrigate the anterior chamber. Triamcinolone adheres to the vitreous and highlights it (Fig. 35.2).

35

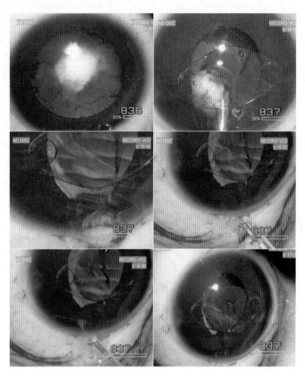

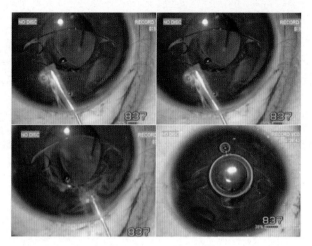

Figure 35.2. The vitreous strands in the anterior chamber are highlighted with triamcinolone and cut with the Fugo blade.

Figure 35.1. The central fibrovascular mass invaded by blood vessels from all sides is cut with a Fugo blade after fixing an iris claw lens. The hyaloid vessel is cut and the fibrovascular mass is removed. The vitreous strands attached to the mass are cut with the Fugo blade outside the incision line.

6. While keeping the anterior chamber deep with visco-elastic material, introduce the Fugo blade under the outlined vitreous, keeping the cutting tip parallel to the iris. Short, sweeping movements of the activated tip cut the vitreous strands instantly.

7. Deal similarly with the fine strands on the iris; this produces no injury to the iris.

8. Perform an iridectomy with a Fugo blade and close the incision line.

Summary

This case illustrates how even a bare-minimum anterior vitrectomy can be performed with the Fugo blade. The procedure requires no aspiration and therefore no traction. The only requirement is clear visualization of the aberrant vitreous, which can be accomplished with triamcinolone irrigation.

Adequate minimum anterior vitrectomy can also be done through the posterior capsulotomy, also without the need for aspiration and traction. Merely touching with and moving the activated Fugo blade tip removes the vitreous.

Suggested Reading

Singh K, Singh SK, Singh IR, et al. Applications of the Fugo blade. *Trop Ophthalmol.* 2007;7:28–36.

Part H
The Posterior Segment

Diabetic Retinopathy INDU R. SINGH

Extraretinal complications of proliferative diabetic retinopathy are caused by neovascular or fibrovascular tissue growth or both, including vitreous hemorrhage, retinal detachment, and other effects that damage the retina or optic nerve. Exact features of fibrovascular tissue growth and secondary complications vary widely from case to case. However, the structural pathogenesis of this disease process is consistent because the abnormal tissue nearly always grows along the posterior vitreous surface.

Different topographic features of proliferative diabetic retinopathy depend on the places of origin and amount of fibrovascular proliferation and the location and extent of any posterior vitreous separation. The location and extent of separation influence the configuration of fibrovascular tissue growth and determine the effect on the underlying and adjacent retina.

Surgical treatment of proliferative diabetic retinopathy is based on this fundamental structural pathophysiology. The principles of surgery are to minimize damaging effects by reversing the optical and structural complications and prevent a recurrence of similar problems.

Therefore, the objectives of surgery are to remove any intravitreal opacities and to excise the posterior vitreous surface. To achieve these objectives, various specialized techniques are required, depending on the complexity of vitreoretinal anatomy in each case.

Surgical Technique

1. Perform a central vitrectomy, clearing the axial opacities and cortical vitreous gel.

2. Create a large opening in the posterior hyaloid until vitreoretinal adhesions are encountered.

3. Perform segmentation or delamination (or both) of these adhesions. One of these procedures is used in virtually all cases of diabetic tractional retinal detachment. Delamination is separation of the retina from extraretinal proliferation from posterior to anterior. In very thick and highly vascular proliferative membranes, the main complication is intra-ocular bleeding. Sometimes this bleeding is so profuse and uncontrollable that it is difficult to save the eye.

We have used the Fugo blade in these cases to cut and close blood vessels at the same time. An example of such a case follows.

CASE STUDY

What follows is a case of proliferative diabetic retinopathy in which complete vitrectomy is done with a vitrector. A large fibrovascular band of tissue was removed using a Fugo blade (Fig. 36.1).

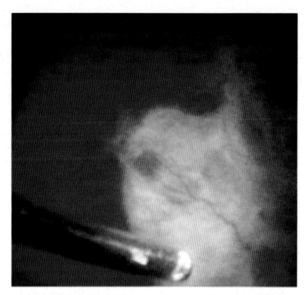

Figure 36.1. Fibrovascular tissue with a sheet of hemorrhage on the retina.

Surgical Technique

1. After an adequate vitrectomy, aspirate the sheet of hemorrhage with a flute needle, exposing the borders of the fibrovascular frond. Use a retinal pick to lift the edge of the membrane (Fig. 36.2).

2. Approach the fibrovascular membrane using an end-gripping forceps in one hand and a Fugo blade tip in the other. We used the OFFISS system of the Topcon microscope to provide endo-illumination.

3. Lift the edge of the membrane slightly off the retinal surface with the end-gripping forceps and apply the Fugo blade tip to the tissue to ablate it. Cavitation bubbles will be seen rising from the site of application (Fig. 36.3).

4. In our case, the procedure progressed slowly, with continued Fugo ablation, regrasping of the tissue, and re-application of the Fugo blade

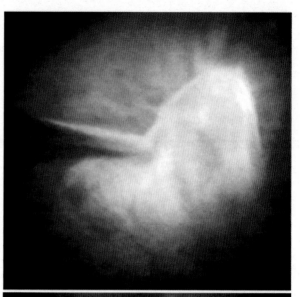

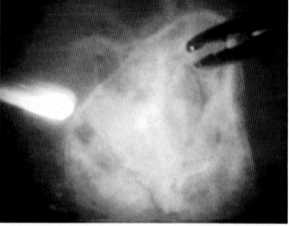

Figure 36.2. Fibrous membrane held with forceps and being cut with the Fugo blade.

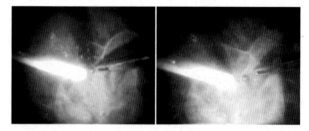

Figure 36.3. Fugo blade ablation in progress.

energy (Fig. 36.4). There was no bleeding from the tissue being treated.

5. A significant portion of the fibrovascular membrane can be cleared off from the retinal surface using just the forceps and the Fugo blade tip. Further lift and incise the fibrovascular membrane with the Fugo blade. When bigger vessels are cut with the Fugo blade, some bleeding can be expected.

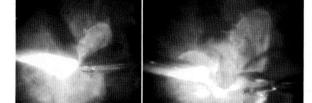

Figure 36.4. Successive stages of membrane being ablated.

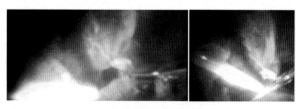

Figure 36.5. Completion of membrane removal.

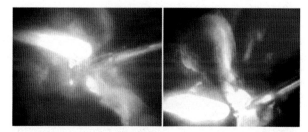

Figure 36.6. Complete membrane removal.

6. Similarly tackle the remainder of the membrane until all of it is removed (Figs. 36.5 and 36.6).

7. After complete removal of the membranes, flatten the retina with perfluorocarbon liquid. To provide a tamponade, endo-laser the retina and fill the vitreous cavity with silicone oil.

Summary

Management of retinal vasoproliferative tissue presents a major challenge for vitreoretinal surgeons. The recent practice of intravitreal injection of an anti–vascular endothelial growth factor agent a few days before vitrectomy has also been helpful in making the surgery a bit easier by reducing intraoperative bleeding. The Fugo blade is a new tool that further enhances the safety profile of this complex surgical procedure.

Suggested Reading

Singh IR. Managing proliferative vitreo-retinopathy with the Fugo blade—a case report. *Trop Ophthalmol.* 2001; 1:24–25.

Singh IR. Vitreo-retinal surgery with plasma blade: a case report. *Trop Ophthalmol.* 2001;1:13–16.

Singh IR, Singh D, Singh RK, et al. The plasma blade in vitreoretinal surgery. *Ann Ophthalmol.* 2001;33:280–289.

37 Encysted Metallic Intra-ocular Foreign Body in the Retina INDU R. SINGH

A case of a metal foreign body impacted in the retina and encysted in thick fibrous tissue is described below.

CASE STUDY

The patient had been injured 8 years previously while hitting tempered steel with a hammer. He had consulted an eye surgeon, who operated on him and declared that the foreign body had been removed. Thereafter, the patient had no further examinations. The patient presented to our clinic when a cataract started to develop. Ocular examination revealed that the foreign body was still present. This was confirmed with B-scan ultrasound and computed tomographic scan.

Surgical Technique

1. For our case, we adopted the standard pars plana vitrectomy technique.

2. After clearing off the dense vitreous haze, we encountered an encysted iron foreign body impacted in the retina, completely surrounded with thick fibrous tissue (Fig. 37.1).

3. During vitrectomy the foreign body was located. It was impacted in the retinal surface but cocooned within a layer of fibrosis that seemed

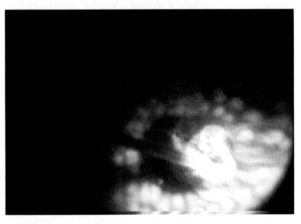

Figure 37.1. Encapsulated metallic foreign body in the retina.

to have enveloped it over the years. The fibrosis was so thick that it could not be opened with the tip of a vitrector or the sharp tip of a 24-gauge needle. We even tried using a diamond blade mounted on a 20-gauge tip to cut the shell open but to no avail. Even with the sharpest diamond blade, you need some counterpressure for the knife to work. We decided to use the Fugo blade. Before using the Fugo blade, however, sufficient endo-laser application was done around the point of impact of the foreign body.

4. A plasma knife tip long enough to reach the retinal surface was used to expose the foreign body (Figs. 37.2 and 37.3).

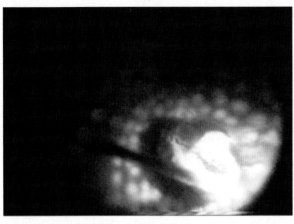

Figure 37.2. Fibrous capsule being cut with the Fugo blade.

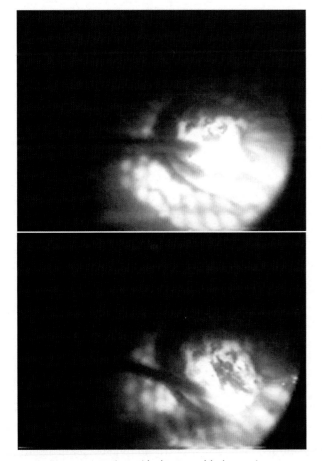

Figure 37.3. Cutting with the Fugo blade continues.

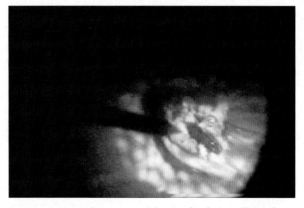

Figure 37.4. The encysted foreign body is sufficiently exposed.

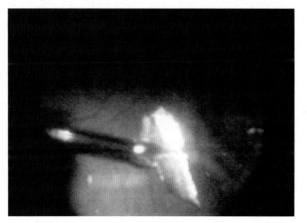

Figure 37.5. The foreign body is extracted from the fibrous capsule.

fibrous shell and out of the eye through the sclerotomy opening (Fig. 37.5).

Summary

Clinical situations such as the case described here may arise only rarely in the course of an ophthalmologist's career. We can think of no other way to successfully manage an encysted metallic foreign body. This case, and its outcome, strengthens our belief that the Fugo blade is a versatile cutting tool that can prove helpful in the most unlikely situations.

Suggested Reading

Singh IR. Managing proliferative vitreo-retinopathy with the Fugo blade—a case report. *Trop Ophthalmol*. 2001; 1:24–25.

Singh IR. Vitreo-retinal surgery with plasma blade: a case report. *Trop Ophthalmol*. 2001;1:13–16.

Singh IR, Singh D, Singh RK, et al. The plasma blade in vitreoretinal surgery. *Ann Ophthalmol*. 2001;33:280–289.

5. In only three to four repetitive passes of the Fugo blade, the encapsulated foreign body was sufficiently exposed (Fig. 37.4). During this process, no push was generated by the plasma knife, as there would be with a needle and a diamond blade.

6. An intraocular foreign body forceps was then used to gently remove the foreign body from the

38 Von Hippel–Lindau Disease

INDU R. SINGH

on Hippel–Lindau disease (VHL) is a genetic condition that involves the growth of angiomas in highly vascular areas of body, including the retina. Although the angioma from VHL can grow in the brain, spinal cord, adrenal glands, kidney, and pancreas, an angioma in the eye is the only VHL hemangioma that can be directly observed.

Pathophysiology and Clinical Presentation

Lesions in VHL can be single or multiple, with considerable variation in appearance and progression through the various stages. Five clinical stages can be identified, as discussed below.

Preclassical

In this stage, small capillary clusters can be seen in the retina. Lesions appear as simple red spots or microaneurysms.

Classical

The classical retinal hemangioma is a knot of vessels with a large artery as a feeder vessel leading to the hemangioma and a large vein as a draining vessel. In the early stages, the hemangioma appears as a nodule with normal-sized vessels. As the lesion grows, the feeder vessels can become two or three times the size of a normal retinal artery or vein. Eventually the lesion becomes elevated. Depending on the location of the lesion, these could be asymptomatic or symptomatic.

Exudative

Fluid leaks across the walls of the lesion result in retinal edema, retinal exudates, and leaked proteins and plasma from the blood. The accumulation of fluid causes retinal swelling and edema. The symptoms may include blurred vision, loss of visual acuity, or vision distortion.

Retinal Detachment

The retinal exudates and edema lift the retina from the choroid. This has a tendency to spread and may cause partial or complete loss of vision.

End Stage

In this stage, the retinal detachment progresses. Glial or scar tissue is likely to form, which may lead to painful glaucoma, and vision maybe permanently lost.

CASE STUDY

We have treated three patients who had stage four VHL with extensive exudates and retinal detachment. One case example is discussed below.

Case

A 48-year-old man presented with no light perception in left eye for 2 years. He gave a history of gradual, painless loss of vision in the left eye for 2 months. On examination, the intra-ocular pressure was low. Examination of the anterior segment showed early cataract changes. Fundus examination of the right eye showed a complicated and old retinal detachment. Fundus examination of the left eye showed a slight media haze with retinal exudation and detachment. At the 5 o'clock position on the periphery lay a circumscribed exophytic retinal capillary hemangioma approximately 2 disc diameter with a prominent dilated and tortuous feeding artery and draining vein (Figs. 38.1–38.4).

All treatment options were discussed in great detail with the patient, including the risks involved and the possibility of uncontrollable bleeding. The

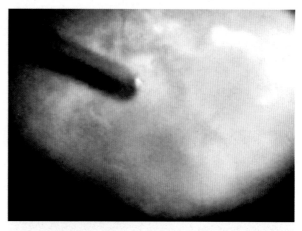

Figure 38.4. The vascular tumor with feeding and draining vessels.

Fugo blade was our instrument of choice for dealing with this tumor.

Surgical Technique

1. Perform a complete pars plana vitrectomy and remove the membranes from the retinal surface with end-gripping forceps.

2. Ablate the tumor with the activated Fugo tip until no sign of it is left (Figs. 38.5 and 38.6). No bleeding from the tumor should occur. The engorged vessels retract and slowly thin.

3. Flatten the retina using perfluorocarbon liquid and then use a laser after releasing the retinal traction from the periphery of the vascular tumor (Fig. 38.7).

4. After settling the retina, inject silicone oil to tamponade the retina.

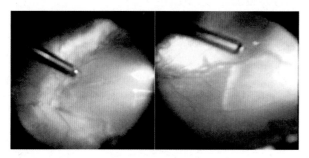

Figure 38.1. Dilated vessels with retinal detachment and exudation.

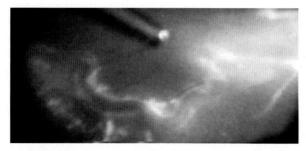

Figure 38.2. Dilated and tortous feeding and draining vessels.

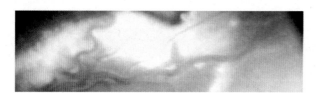

Figure 38.3. Extensive subretinal exudation.

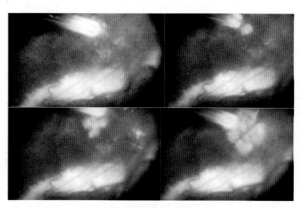

Figure 38.5. Direct ablation of the vascular tumor with the Fugo blade. No bleeding is present.

38

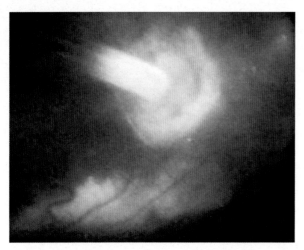

Figure 38.6. Nearly completed tumor ablation.

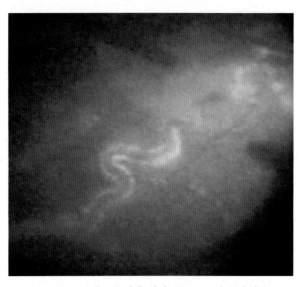

Figure 38.7. Subretinal fluid drainage and endo-laser were applied around the vascular tumor. The large vessels connected to the tumor have shrunk.

Postoperative Management

Postoperatively, our patient was followed for 4 months before the silicone oil was removed. The patient recovered with 6/24 vision.

Because there was no tumor left, blood vessels supplying the area lost their tortuosity and diminished in size. All that remained of the tumor was a dense white scar in the periphery.

Summary

This surgery is generally not attempted for fear of bleeding from the engorged vessels of Von Hippel–Lindau disease and the tumor, but the Fugo blade made this procedure simple and safe.

Suggested Reading

Singh IR. Managing proliferative vitreo-retinopathy with the Fugo blade—a case report. *Trop Ophthalmol.* 2001;1:24–25.

Singh IR. Vitreo-retinal surgery with plasma blade: a case report. *Trop Ophthalmol.* 2001;1:13–16.

Singh IR, Singh D, Singh RK, et al. The plasma blade in vitreoretinal surgery. *Ann Ophthalmol.* 2001;33:280–289.

Eales Disease INDU R. SINGH

E ales disease is an idiopathic obliterative vasculopathy that usually involves the peripheral retina in young adults. In 1880, Henry Eales first described it in healthy young men with abnormal retinal veins and recurrent vitreous hemorrhages.

Clinical findings are characterized by avascular areas in the retinal periphery, followed posteriorly by microaneurysms, dilatation of capillary channels, tortuosity of neighboring vessels, and spontaneous chorioretinal scars. It is a diagnosis of exclusion, as many other retinal disorders can mimic Eales disease, especially conditions of retinal inflammation or neovascularization.

Pathophysiology and Clinical Presentation

The pathophysiology of Eales disease is mostly unknown. It is believed to be a primary, noninflammatory disorder of the walls of peripheral retinal vessels that often leads to vascular occlusions, peripheral neovascularization, and vitreous hemorrhage. The microvascular abnormalities are seen at the junction of perfused and nonperfused zones of the retina.

Patients often present with symptoms of floaters, cobwebs, and blurring or decreased vision associated with vitreous hemorrhage. Clinical findings usually involve the retina and the vitreous. Vascular sheathing and hemorrhages of the adjacent nerve fiber layer are the most common findings. The sheathing can range from mild to severe to causing vascular occlusions. Areas of vascular sheathing often leak on fluorescein angiography.

Anterior chamber and vitreous may exhibit cell flare and keratitic precipitates. Cystoid macular edema may occur because of low-grade inflammation. Epiretinal membranes are also a frequent occurrence.

Peripheral nonperfusion is a typical feature of Eales disease. The surrounding vasculature is tortuous with microvascular abnormalities, which include microaneurysms, arteriovenous shunts, venous beading, hard exudates, and cotton-wool spots. Fine solid white lines occasionally can be seen, indicating obliterated larger vessels.

Branch retinal-vein occlusion (BRVO) can be seen in patients with Eales disease; it may be limited to one area or may be multifocal, unlike BRVO alone, which is usually confined to a single affected quadrant and respects the anatomical distribution of the horizontal raphe.

Neovascularization of the disc (NVD) or neovascularization elsewhere (NVE) in the retina is observed in up to 80% of patients with Eales disease. The NVE usually is located peripherally, at the junction of perfused and nonperfused retina. Neovascularization is often the source of vitreous hemorrhage in these eyes. Rubeosis iridis, or neovascularization of the iris, can develop and may lead to neovascular glaucoma. Fibrovascular proliferation on the surface of the retina may accompany retinal neovascularization. These eyes have associated anteroposterior traction that could lead to retinal detachment.

CASE STUDY

The patient had Eales disease with NVD, NVE, and retinal traction, and pars plana vitrectomy was performed to clear the vitreous hemorrhage and to clear

39

the fibrovascular proliferative tissue created by the disease (Fig. 39.1).

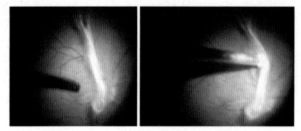

Figure 39.1. A fibrovascular band extends from the disc to the periphery. A vitrectomy cutter was abandoned in favor of a Fugo blade because it created traction on the macula.

Surgical Technique

1. In our case, we first tried to use a vitrector to cut the band, but it created traction on the macula, so we abandoned this approach. We decided to use the Fugo blade to cut this band. For this purpose, an elongated 20-gauge Fugo tip was used because it could negotiate the 20-gauge sclerotomies and was long enough to reach the retina (Fig. 39.2).

2. Activate the Fugo blade tip and start cutting by merely touching the tissue. No traction is produced while cutting. Cavitation bubbles will be seen while the band is being cut (Figs. 39.2 and 39.3).

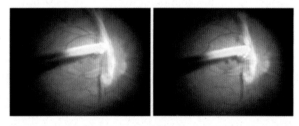

Figure 39.2. The Fugo blade tip is activated and touched to the lesion.

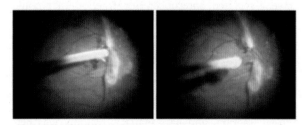

Figure 39.3. The proliferative band is bisected.

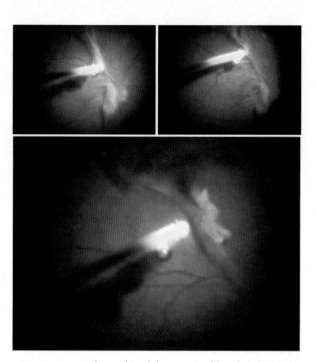

Figure 39.4. The stubs of the vasoproliferative tissue are ablated.

3. After bisecting the band, direct the Fugo blade to ablate the stubs of the band toward their attachment points on the retina (Fig. 39.4).

4. Remove the stubs of the vasoproliferative tissue with a combination of a vitreous cutter, endo-scissors, and endo-forceps.

5. During this process, the only difficulty we encountered was that the cavitation bubbles rose up and made it hard to see the surgical field. We had to aspirate the bubbles often when they affected visibility beyond a certain point.

Summary

Although this case is of one of Eales disease, similar pathologic pictures of varying severity are seen in other diseases and similarly result in proliferative fibrovascular tissues. The Fugo blade is excellent in managing complex proliferative tissues.

Suggested Reading

Singh IR. Managing proliferative vitreo-retinopathy with the Fugo blade—a case report. *Trop Ophthalmol.* 2001;1: 13–16.

Singh IR, Singh D, Singh RK, et al. The plasma blade in vitreoretinal surgery. *Ann Ophthalmol.* 2001;33:12–20.

Part I
The Cornea

Pterygium Surgery DALJIT SINGH

T he pterygium may be operated on in many ways, but in each case, it must be removed from its bed and excised. Recurrent pterygia are more difficult to treat because of the extensive scar tissue that is firmly rooted in the sclera. In recurrent cases, the involved corneal tissue is also firmly attached to the thick scar tissue.

In the "bare sclera" technique for pterygium surgery the cornea should be fully cleared of the pterygium, and no raised area should be near the limbus for a distance of 3 to 5 mm. I have been using this technique for most of my surgical career.

Whenever tissue must be removed, the question arises whether it should be removed with the standard forceps scissors and bipolar tools or the new ablative tool, the Fugo blade. For a while I used the Fugo blade to assist in removing excessive scar tissue during a mainly manual excision of the pterygium. Gradually, however, my technique for pterygium removal has increasingly involved use of the Fugo blade. A description follows.

TECHNIQUE

Anesthesia

Provide surface anesthesia with 2% lidocaine.

Surgical Technique

1. Open the conjunctiva with a 100-μm Fugo blade tip, near the upper edge of the pterygium, about 1 mm from the limbus. To minimize the risk of subconjunctival bleeding, do not use a needle. Instead, inject lignocaine through the opening under the conjunctiva with a 30-gauge cannula. Advance the cannula toward the lower edge of the pterygium, where it is used to lift the conjunctiva. Some subconjunctival bleeding may be seen as the blunt cannula is advanced (Fig. 40.1).

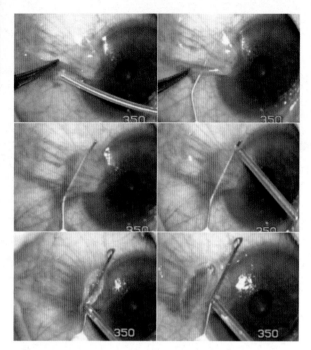

Figure 40.1. The conjunctiva is opened at the edge of the pterygium with a Fugo blade tip. A cannula injects lignocaine and is advanced to lift the conjunctiva. The conjunctiva is incised in a straight line over the cannula using the 600-μm Fugo blade tip.

2. Touch a 600-μm Fugo blade tip to the conjunctival tent just created by the cannula, so that the cannula tip is bared. Then lift the conjunctiva over the cannula. Ablate the lifted conjunctiva from the tip upward until it comes free and falls off (Fig. 40.2).

3. Peel the pterygium from the cornea with forceps alone or with assistance from the 600-μm Fugo blade tip. If the corneal surface appears rough, smooth it by rubbing the Fugo blade tip over the roughness. Do the smoothing under a stream of saline, not over dry cornea.

4. Touch any bleeding point on the sclera with the 600-μm Fugo blade tip. Also, move the tip under the cut edge of the conjunctiva to control any blood ooze. Normally, I do not touch the delicate vessels over the sclera, but in this particular case I was tempted to ablate a large vessel. It is prudent not to touch the normal vasculature. Therefore, blanching the sclera with a bipolar cautery or with the Fugo blade is not desirable.

5. Use blunt scissors to undermine the cut edge of the conjunctiva to free it from possibly abnormal subconjunctival tissue. The Fugo blade cut of the conjunctiva has a clean margin and although it is cut in a straight line, it will automatically curve as it retracts from the cornea.

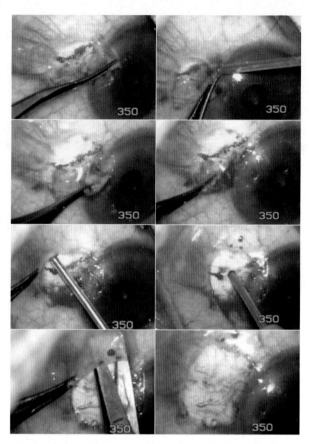

Figure 40.2. A pterygium is peeled off with partial assistance from the Fugo blade. The cut edge of the conjunctiva is undermined with the 600-μm Fugo blade tip and blunt scissors. Any bleeder on the surface of the sclera is also ablated.

6. Do not use mitomycin after surgery. We are aware of five cases in which scleral necrosis developed after mitomycin was administered. (No data was available on the concentration of mitomycin used or its duration.)

7. In recurrent and complicated cases it is best to save as much of the conjunctiva as possible. If the bare scleral area is large, undermine the conjunctival edge and bring it forward and suture it to the sclera (Fig. 40.3). Another option is to place an amniotic membrane graft on the bare sclera.

8. A straight-line Fugo blade cut in the conjunctiva is an excellent preparation for excision of a pterygium. Its closeness to the limbus varies from case to case. Remove scar tissue over the cornea and the sclera with a 600-μm Fugo blade tip under a stream of saline; this results in a smooth surface.

9. In recurrent cases, apply a bandage lens at the end of the surgery and remove it after 2 weeks.

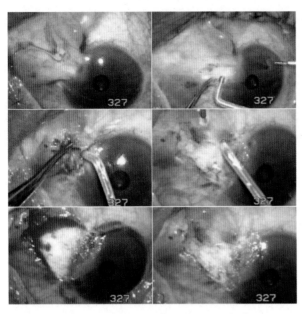

Figure 40.3. Management of a severe case of recurrent pterygium. The scar tissue has been removed with the Fugo blade and the sclera bared. The conjunctival edge has been advanced and sutured to the sclera.

Postoperative Management

Remove the pad 3 hours after the surgery. Prescribe for the patient to use antibiotic–steroid ointment three times a day for 15 days. Starting 1 day after surgery, use mitomycin 2 mg mixed in 5 ml of artificial tear drops four times a day for 7 days. The potency of mitomycin declines rapidly. This formulation of mitomycin has not resulted in any case of scleral necrosis. Only one to two re-operations a year have been done at our clinic. The rate is quite low considering that over 500 operations are done every year.

Summary

Pterygium excision with the Fugo blade results in a nice scleral surface with an intact natural pattern of blood vessels (Fig. 40.4). Together with a clean semi-circular cut of the conjunctiva, they provide a very suitable bed on which to put an amniotic graft or an auto-conjunctival graft. The graft may be fixed in place with sutures or with tissue glue.

The Fugo blade is an excellent supplementary tool in any surgical approach to a primary or recurrent pterygium of any severity.

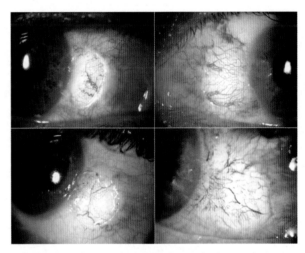

Figure 40.4. Examples of results of the bare sclera technique using the Fugo blade, 3 hours after surgery.

41 Corneal Ulcers DALJIT SINGH

efractory corneal ulcers can sometimes take months to heal. In such cases, corneal transplantation shorten the course of the disease. However, keratoplasty is not possible in some situations, because of either a lack of adequate facilities or the unsuitability of the case. It is also important to rule out predisposing factors, such as diabetes mellitus and immunodeficiency.

Corneal healing requires a clean base over which the epithelium can grow and adhere to firmly cover the gap. Sometimes necrotic tissue adheres to the healthy cornea. Infection may be present, but local anti-infective agents may fail to reach the infected site. Oral medication then becomes the sole agent that may control infection to some extent. Medication and infection may come to a standoff, making no further progress in either direction.

On its own, the body's removal of dead tissue might take weeks or months, in which case the dead tissue/detritus/callus is slowly undermined and broken up by the growing epithelium. But to hasten the healing process, necrotic material must be removed. Cleaning the debris from the corneal ulcer is a serious and delicate process, with the ever-present risk that lurking infection may flare up.

The Fugo blade is useful in managing corneal ulcers.

CASE STUDIES

Case 1: Corneal Ulcer in Uncontrolled Diabetes

A 55-year-old diabetic female patient had a nonhealing corneal ulcer with a hypopyon. She had been under treatment with antibiotics and antifungal agents for over 4 months. A large round central area, the "callus,"

was firmly adhered to the underlying cornea. This was her only cyc. The patient also suffered from severe cardiac and renal problems. Her diabetes remained uncontrolled despite treatment. We opted to remove the callus as a first step to further treatment (Fig. 41.1).

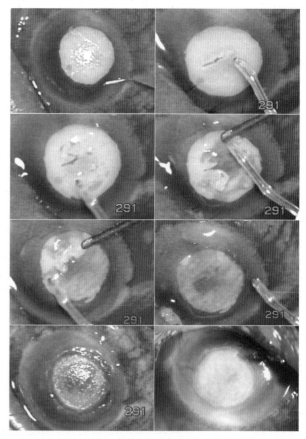

Figure 41.1. The callus is removed under a stream of saline with a 600-μm Fugo blade tip. The final image is the same patient 1 day after surgery.

Surgical Technique

1. In our case, we first used a hockey-stick knife to abrade the callus. The callus felt gritty. No progress was made after two attempts with the hockey-stick knife.

2. We then used a Fugo blade tip at low power and low intensity, but also without success. We realized that it was because the lesion was completely dry.

3. We wetted the cornea and ablated it with the Fugo blade and saw instant results. The callus disappeared in a few seconds. A seemingly healthy cornea appeared from the underneath.

4. We placed a bandage lens on the cornea.

Postoperative Management

Local antibiotic and antifungal drops and artificial tears were used postoperatively. It took almost 2 months for the epithelium to cover half of the ulcer. The patient was able to find her way around her home with her little improvement in vision. That was the last information we had on this patient.

Summary

This case demonstrates the utility of the Fugo blade for cleaning corneal ulcers. It is important to note, however, that the ablating tip should be kept moving at all times under a stream of fluid. Avoid using the Fugo blade when the cornea is very thin.

As with mechanical methods, Fugo blade ablation can make the cornea vulnerable to infection flare-up. Frequent local medication is necessary during the early postoperative period. Eye drops should be used even overnight.

Shield Ulcers

Shield ulcers are common in some patients with severe spring catarrh. The allergy may manifest at the limbus, on the palpebral conjunctiva, or in both places. In every case of shield ulcer, eversion of the lid reveals the classic raised knob or multiple cobblestones. These knobs or cobblestones feel like stones as they press on or rub over the soft cornea. This results in epithelial abrasion, which appears as an elongated ulcer that may look clean, but usually harbors dead, white

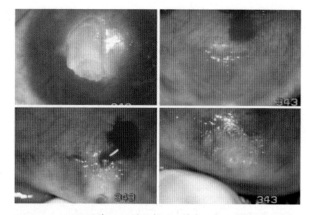

Figure 41.2. A large raised, round, hard nodule, the causative factor in a shield ulcer, is exposed by everting the upper lid. The nodule is rubbed with 600-μm Fugo blade tip until the tarsal lesion becomes flat or even concave.

adherent tissue in the floor. These ulcers do not heal unless the allergy subsides on its own or is treated. In tandem with systemic treatment of the allergy by a specialist, the corneal lesion has to be spared recurrent trauma and pressure from the palpebral lesions.

Manual removal of the palpebral lesions is difficult and accompanied by heavy bleeding. Electrocautery is also traumatic and causes a severe postoperative reaction. The tarsal lesions remain untouched for long periods. The usual approach is to control them with local and systemic steroids.

The Fugo blade is very useful in these cases (Fig. 41.2). Anesthesia consists of everting the lid and injecting lignocaine along the upper edge of the tarsal plate. A single lesion can be decimated in a few seconds. The plethora of cobblestones can be managed as described below.

Surgical Technique

1. Expose the palpebral conjunctiva with an everter.

2. Use a 600-μm Fugo blade tip at high power and high energy. Treat each cobblestone with one, two, or more pushes of the activated tip. The tip removes the bulk from these hard nodules and flattens them.

3. Do not touch the areas between the nodules. The whole process is complete in just a few minutes.

4. At the end of surgery, inject dilute triamcinolone along the whole breadth of the conjunctiva, along the upper edge of the tarsal plate (Fig. 41.3). Patients with shield ulcers from spring allergies should be followed by both an ophthalmologist and an allergist.

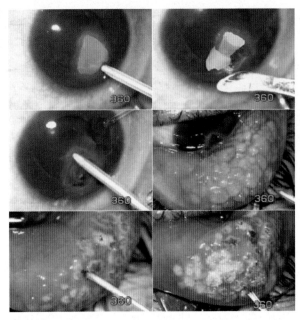

Figure 41.3. The Fugo blade had no effect on the dry callus on this shield ulcer; the callus was removed mechanically. However, the base was cleaned with the Fugo blade and individual cobblestones were "debulked" with Fugo blade ablation.

Suggested Reading

Guttman C. Anterior segment tool proves ideal for many applications. *Ophthalmol Times.* 2005;30:14–16.

McGrath D. Fugo blade effective tool for multiple surgical applications. *Eurotimes.* 2008;13:43.

Winn CW. Broad applications seen for electrosurgical instrument. *Ocular Surg News.* 2001;19:45–46.

Corneal Edema DALJIT SINGH

42

F or the cornea to maintain hydration, transparency, and metabolism, fluid must move throughout the stroma. But does the fluid move because of diffusion only between the stroma and the limiting membranes on both sides, or is there a more efficient channel system? Is the cornea kept transparent by simple dehydration or hydration only, or is there a more efficient system that handles the cornea's metabolic requirements? For all practical purposes, the cornea is transparent, so it is difficult to visualize any channels that may run through it.

My colleagues and I have been studying the conjunctival lymphatics for many years. We have demonstrated conjunctival lymphatics by injecting trypan blue under the distal subconjunctival area. Further research revealed that injecting the dye in the peripheral cornea, rather than in the subconjunctival area, made the lymphatics even more apparent. We also tried to chart lymphatics in the cornea. To demonstrate channels in the cornea, we injected trypan blue in the corneal stroma close to the limbus in painful blind eyes undergoing glaucoma surgery. A small ball of the dye could be created locally. At the edges of the ball, small projections of the dye were visible toward the center and the periphery, but there was whitening of the cornea due to pressure from the injected fluid. Slit-lamp examination did not show positive proof that the dye was moving toward the center, but the dye did disappear toward the periphery within a few days, proving that at least centrifugal fluid movement in the cornea was present. Visualization of the corneal channels has not yet been documented.

At one point, while studying pictures of conjunctival lymphatics, I found that the dye that had filled them had also created a thin circular line in the periphery of the

cornea. The line could not be the Schlemm canal, because it was anterior to the angle of the anterior chamber (Fig. 42.1). On another occasion, during an enucleation procedure, dye was injected with great force into the cornea some distance from the limbus. The dye filled a ring-like space along the limbus (Fig. 42.2).

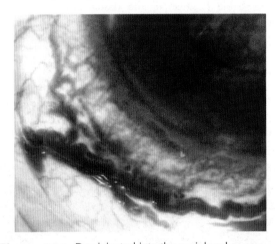

Figure 42.1. Dye injected into the peripheral cornea demonstrated not only the conjunctival lymphatics but also a blue arc in the corneal periphery.

One would expect any form of invisible corneal channels, if present, to be transparent and similar to sinusoids, rather than definitive vessels like arteries and veins. But suppose a corneal pathology renders the corneal tissue translucent or semi-opaque, thus making the channels visible, just as the transparent limbal lymphatics become visible when slight pigment is around them?

This possibility occurred to me when I first saw a young patient with keratoglobus who had an opacity in the center of the cornea. Prominent networklike,

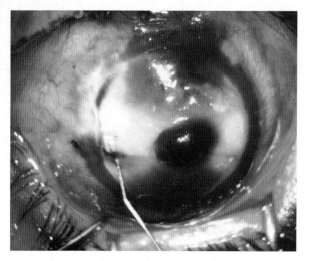

Figure 42.2. Trypan blue injected into the cornea has assumed a circular form inside the limbus.

channels are in the corneal stroma. The appearance is not attributable to changes in the Descemet membrane. How does so much postoperative keratitis/edema disappear in a matter of hours or days? This probably occurs because the channels in the cornea act like flood drains, as they do elsewhere in the body (Fig. 42.4).

We soon learned that the best place to study corneal channels is the area in and around the arcus senilis. The semi-opacification of the arcus highlights the channels. The pattern of the channels is practically the same as in the case of keratoglobus described above. The channels go right up to the lucid interval of arcus senilis. Many of the network channels terminate in the lucid interval, which is lucid seemingly because it has more sinusoidal channels than elsewhere. An optical section of a lucid interval shows a

darkish lines divided the large nebular corneal opacity into many geometrical compartments. The lines were nearly uniform in size and became fainter and then disappeared toward the transparent peripheral cornea. They did not appear to be any kind of pathology, but were visible because of the tissue changes around them. On optical section they were seen to be in the stroma. The endothelial side was normal. We have been watching this patient for over 9 years; his corneal condition remains the same (Fig. 42.3).

A case of postoperative striate keratitis also sheds light on the existence of the corneal channels. Corneal edema is present, and some sort of channel network is visible. Optical section shows that the

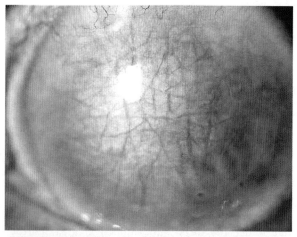

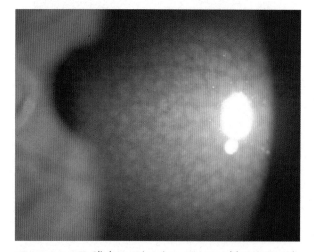

Figure 42.3. Slit-lamp view in a 10-year-old patient with megalocornea. A network of channels is visible in the central and paracentral parts of the cornea. The flashlight could highlight only a part of the opacity.

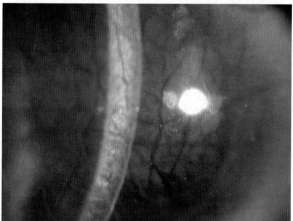

Figure 42.4. A case of severe striate keratitis showing island formation due to the appearance of a network of corneal channels. The optical section shows that they are located in the deep corneal stroma. They also show anterior connections.

42

roughly triangular shape, with the base toward the periphery and semi-opaque plates of the corneal tissue on both sides (Figs. 42.5–42.7).

It is probably that even finer channels have so far escaped our notice. If we examine cases of nondescript

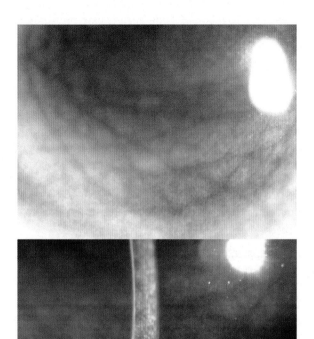

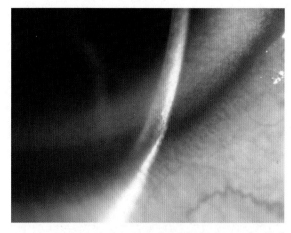

Figure 42.7. Optical section through the corneal periphery. The arcus senilis shows a prominent lucid interval. Fine channels in the arcus and lymphatics at the edge of the lucid interval are also visible.

keratitis under high magnification, we see very fine feathery structures. If these are the finest branches of the corneal sinusoidal channels, they could permeate elements of the corneal tissue (Fig. 42.8).

Fluid flows from the cornea in myriad lymphatic channels in the limbus. Their corneal ends disappear into the corneal periphery and their proximal ends merge into the conjunctival lymphatics. It is not far-fetched to say that continuity exists between the corneal sinusoidal system and the limbal and conjunctival lymphatics. One can liken the eyeball to a sponge, with the porosity of the channels varying from one tissue to the next. We have been trained to study the tissues histopathologically. When we do not find a

Figure 42.5. A profusion of large and small network channels in an 82-year-old patient. Optical section shows that the wider channels are situated in the deeper layers and that they have connections anteriorly.

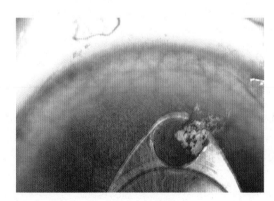

Figure 42.6. Network of corneal channels. Notice a periodic merging of the channels into the lucid interval.

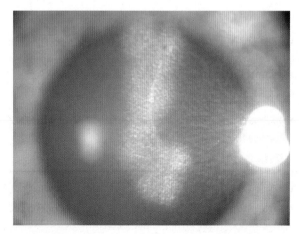

Figure 42.8. The finest chinks in the corneal structure are visible in this particular form of stromal keratitis.

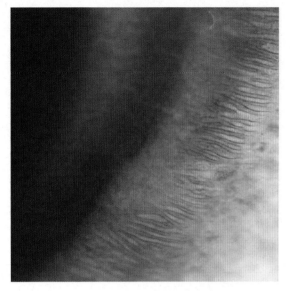

Figure 42.9. Numerous lymphatics appear over the arcus senilis and at the edge of the lucid interval.

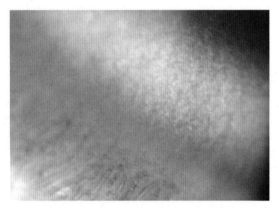

Figure 42.10. The relationship between the limbal lymphatics and channels in lucid interval and arcus senilis.

structure, it is supposed not to exist. At present, the corneal channels can be studied only in vivo under a slit-lamp microscope (Figs. 42.9 and 42.10).

Relationship to the Intra-ocular Aqueous

When such a dense network exists close to the limbus right on top of the Schlemm canal, it is inconceivable that connections do not exist between them. We do not have photographic proof of interconnecting channels, but we have a clinical situation that points to the existence of that connection, as discussed below.

The cornea becomes edematous in cases of acute glaucoma. The moment the pressure is released by paracentesis, the cornea clears up within seconds. This change could not occur without the assumed channels and their connections to the source of raised intra-ocular pressure. Why do many advanced cases of open-angle glaucoma, with intra-ocular pressures as high as 50 mm Hg or greater, not show corneal edema? It is possible that the channels system has been adapting and increasing the flow along the channels, so that the cornea remains transparent, while the optic disc continues to excavate.

Also, what is the function of limbal capillaries? Do they function the way they function in the rest of the body? We imagine a regular formation of lymph around the cornea that nourishes it through a network of channels. Following this theory, then, fluid movement is dynamic activity, making the cornea a living and throbbing entity, rather than a piece of transparent tissue.

Corneal Decompensation

Fluids do not stay still in the body, and the cornea is no exception. Every heartbeat moves fluids throughout the body. Fluid loads increase or fluid movement is retarded by local causes, and these manifest as edema or decompensation. The presence of edema reduces the transfer of oxygen toward the endothelium, further damaging the endothelium. When the endothelium is at fault, this vicious cycle has to be broken; the standard solution is a full-thickness corneal graft.

In many situations, a corneal graft is either not available or is not performed for personal, social, or medical reasons. At such times, it is possible to help the patient by making new channels to improve or increase drainage of the cornea. Vertical ablation channels/pits are made with the help of the Fugo blade. These ablation pits drain the posterior layers of the cornea toward the anterior layers; from there the fluid is picked up by the more superficial drainage channels and carried to the limbal–conjunctival system and ultimately to the general circulation.

Ablation Pits for Corneal Edema

Management by creating ablation pits is indicated in cases of bullous or nonbullous keratopathy resulting from corneal decompensation, when either corneal graft material is not available or the patient is medically unfit for corneal graft surgery or cannot afford it. The technique is described below.

TECHNIQUE

The corneal thickness is visually estimated on optical section with a slit-lamp microscope. The more sophisticated methods are pachymetry and optical coherence tomography. This is important because a proper length of Fugo blade ablating tip is required in order to avoid the danger of perforation during surgery. A 100-μm tip, about 350 to 400 mm long is selected for surgery. The chosen tip is bent to meet the ergonomic needs of the surgeon.

Anesthesia

Topical anesthesia is enough for this surgery.

Surgical Technique

1. Creation of the pit with the Fugo blade starts at the periphery of the cornea. Make 8 to 12 pits close the limbus. Because the Fugo blade tip has a stopper at the preselected length, the danger of perforation is avoided. Select medium power and energy settings. A pit is instantly created as the activated tip is pressed into the cornea.
2. Make the second row of ablation pits inside the outer row.
3. Make the third row approaching the edge of the pupil. Leave the pupillary area untouched.

Some patients have thick scarred epithelium loosely attached to the corneal stroma. In such cases the epithelium should be removed. Keep in mind the remaining thickness of the cornea mind when dealing with such a case.

CASE STUDIES

Case 1

This 85-year-old, very poor patient traveled over a thousand miles to see me, some 18 years after I had implanted an intra-ocular lens in his remaining seeing eye. This time, the patient presented with a frank case of corneal decompensation. The only conceivable treatment was a full-thickness corneal graft. However, I did not have a suitable facility to perform the procedure, nor was there one available anywhere in the state. Regardless, the patient could not have afforded it anywhere because of his inability to pay.

At the time, I was looking into the concept of corneal channels. By this time, too, I had had 2 years of experience using the Fugo blade. I knew that it would ablate tissues without collateral damage. The patient and I were in a hopeless situation. I thought: Why not try draining the cornea with Fugo blade pits? I explained my plan to the patient and his grandson, and both agreed readily.

First we tried hypertonic saline every 2 minutes for 1 hour. The cornea cleared to some extent, but it was obvious that not much could be achieved through this approach, so we went ahead with the ablation pit approach.

Surgery was done by making multiple pits in the cornea as described above. The cornea appeared somewhat clear 4 hours after surgery. Hypertonic drops were instilled every hour. On the 5th day after surgery the condition was even better. By the 10th day after surgery, the patient could walk about freely without assistance. The endothelial-cell count 10 days after surgery was 458 cells per cubic millimeter, as determined using a Bioptics (high-powered microscope) contact-type specular endothelial microscope.

We sent the patient home and requested that he return after 2 months, if possible. His health was not good and I expected never to see him again. However, he did return, and we were delighted with what we saw. He had a perfectly clear cornea in which the position of Fugo blade pits was marked by gray spots. His corrected vision was 6/12. The endothelial-cell count had risen to 980 cells per cubic millimeter. He kept coming for 4 more years. Transparency of the cornea and good vision persisted, and his endothelial-cell counts hovered around 1000 cells per cubic millimeter (Fig. 42.11).

Case 2

A 70-year-old patient presented with full-blown corneal decompensation after about 20 years of lens implant surgery. Treatment corneal pits made with the Fugo blade resolved the edema in about 3 months. Her best vision was 6/6 and the endothelial-cell count was 680 cells per cubic millimeter (Fig. 42.12). She did not return to the clinic.

Summary

Over the past 6 years we have performed this corneal pit treatment on more than 40 patients with all grades of corneal decompensation severity. Regardless of the cause of the condition, every patient has improved to some extent, and a few to a great extent. Pain and

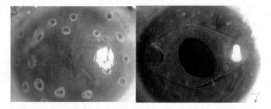

Figure 42.12. A 70-year-old patient (Case 2) with corneal decompensation 1 day and 3 months after surgery.

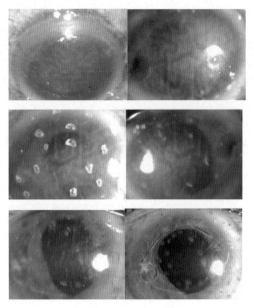

Figure 42.11. This 85-year-old patient with corneal decompensation (Case 1) improved slightly with hypertonic saline. Fugo blade pits on the 1st, 5th, and 10th days after surgery show rapid improvement. The last image, taken 2 months after surgery, shows complete clearing of the cornea. The marks of the Fugo blade tip are visible.

grittiness lessened or disappeared in cases of bullous keratopathy. Corneal edema is reduced or completely disappears, with consequent improvement in vision. Patients' visual improvement has been constant over years of follow-up. Endothelial-cell counts have risen as the corneal condition improves. Some patients have been treated more than once. Depending on the visual demands of the patient, he or she can be referred for cornea transplantation at any time. Fugo blade pits do not interfere with any kind of corneal procedure.

It is a common belief that the number of endothelial cells is fixed. This is most probably not true. Real life is more dynamic. We have seen endothelial-cell counts increase after patients stop using contact lenses and after removing lenses supporting dislocated irises. Using a Bioptics contact type specular endothelial microscope, we have seen evidence of amitotic cell division close to the site of endothelial injury. We have studied the corneal endothelium immediately after photorefractive keratectomy and in the following days. The endothelial damage increases with increasing degrees of refractive error treated. The process of repair and recovery starts soon. During this period, we frequently see evidence of amitotic cell division. It seems that endothelial-cell recovery plays an important part in the improvements noted after treating corneal decompensation with Fugo blade pits.

Fugo blade pits are made in a matter of minutes. Little medication is required after surgery, and immune complications present no risk, as with corneal grafts. This treatment and its great benefits can be extended to every patient for whom a corneal graft is not possible.

Suggested Reading

Singh D, et al. The conjunctival lymphatic system. *Ann Ophthalmol.* 2003;35:99–104.

Dermoid of the Limbus DALJIT SINGH

Dermoids are solid congenital tumors consisting of mesoblastic tissue covered by ectoderm and invaded by ectodermal derivatives. Dermoids may be small and superficial or large and likely deeper within the tissue. They may be located anywhere along the limbus, but they appear most commonly in the lower temporal quadrant. They are not uncommon. Because they are located on a vital thin corneal–scleral tissue and tend to grow over time, dermoids are best recognized and treated early.

Three approaches to managing dermoids are excision, excision with keratectomy, and excision with lamellar keratoplasty. The choice of surgery depends on the needs of the patient, the surgeon's armamentarium and experience, and the availability of donor corneas. The aim of excision is total or subtotal removal of the dermoid, and it is done in such a way as to avoid perforating the cornea. The excision should be smooth enough so that the raw tissue can be covered with epithelium fairly quickly. We have been using the Fugo blade as one of the tools in excision. Two methods are described below.

TECHNIQUE

Anesthesia

Administer general anesthesia.

Surgical Technique

1. For conjunctival tissue covering the dermoid:
   Puncture the conjunctiva covering the dermoid near the limbus with a 100-μm Fugo tip. Balloon the subconjunctiva with saline through a thin cannula. (Not using a needle for this purpose prevents subconjunctival hemorrhage.) See Figure 43.1.

2. Incise the corneal edge of the dermoid with a 100-μm Fugo blade tip kept parallel to the cornea.

3. Continue dissection toward the sclera, removing the middle and anterior bulk of the dermoid.

4. Then cautiously remove the deeper layers, removing ever-finer slices each time. The corneal tissues will become visible. Determine the thickness of the underlying cornea by pressing with the tip of a forceps.

5. Then remove the last remnants of the dermoid over the cornea as follows. Lift the finest layer with the tip of a needle and carry it toward the corneal edge of the lesion, which is excised along with it.

6. Smooth the rough corneal and the scleral edges of the dissection with a 600-μm Fugo blade tip. Keep the activated tip moving under a stream of saline.

7. Straighten the edge of the saved conjunctiva and sutured it at the limbus. Leave the raw area of the cornea alone to heal.

   1. For a dermoid devoid of conjunctival tissue, but with its skin (with or without hair): Balloon the conjunctiva around the dermoid. Incise it with a 100-μm Fugo blade tip and then elevate the conjunctiva with blunt scissors.

   2. Slice the dermoid with the Fugo blade. When more than half the thickness has been removed, use a scissors to remove the strip along the perimeter of the dermoid, including the strip on the cornea as well as on the sclera.

   3. Close any bleeding vessels with a 600-μm Fugo blade tip, operating under a stream of

43

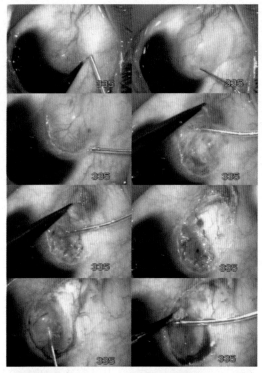

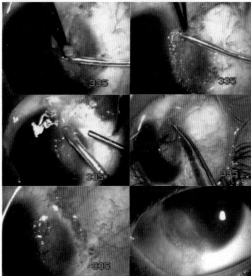

saline, finally obtaining a smooth surface on the cornea as well as on the sclera.

4. Bring the undermined conjunctiva forward and suture it to the sclera as close to the limbus as possible. In less than 2 weeks, the raw area will be covered by the epithelial tissue (Fig. 43.2).

In our case of a limbal dermoid, scissors and Fugo blade tips were combined to remove the limbal dermoid efficiently and with minimum trauma.

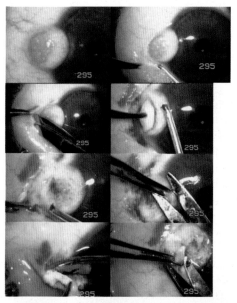

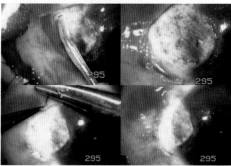

Figure 43.1. Dermoid excision in a 24-year-old patient. The conjunctival covering is ballooned, incised at the corneal end, lifted along with a bulk of the dermoid, and excised with the Fugo blade. The rest of the dermoid mass is excised carefully with the Fugo blade. The base is polished with 600-μm Fugo blade tip under a stream of saline. The conjunctival edge is trimmed, brought forward, and sutured at the limbus. The final image shows the condition of the eye 6 months after surgery.

Figure 43.2. Dermoid excision in a 9-month-old patient. The conjunctiva is ballooned with saline and incised along the edge. Slices of the dermoid are removed, followed by excision at the edges with a scissors. The base of the dermoid over the sclera and the cornea is polished by a 600-μm Fugo blade. The conjunctiva is brought forward and sutured close to the limbus.

Postoperative Management

In all cases of dermoid excision, have the patient apply antibiotic–steroid ointment three times a day. The cornea will be covered with epithelium in about 2 weeks.

The final image in Figure 43.1 shows the condition of our patient's eye 6 months later. There was no change in the best corrected vision of 6/18. The growing lesion is gone. If and when further cosmetic treatment is desired, tattooing or lamellar corneal grafting is available.

Summary

Every effort should be made to remove limbal dermoids completely. The last traces of dermoid tissue can be erased using a 600-μm Fugo blade tip. For those who like to simultaneously graft an amniotic membrane or to do a lamellar keratoplasty, the Fugo blade creates a smooth base for further treatment.

Suggested Reading

Mohan M, Mukherjee G, Panda A. Clinical evaluation and surgical intervention of limbal dermoid. *J All India Ophthalmol Soc.* 1981;29:69–73.

Part J
The Sclera

44 Keratoprosthesis Surgery INDU R. SINGH

Blindness due to corneal disease is usually difficult or impossible to treat. Results of penetrating keratoplasty may be acceptable for classical indications, but in complicated situations such as profusely vascularized corneal opacities, severe ocular surface disorders, or pseudocornea, penetrating keratoplasty is either not indicated or not possible. In such cases, the only possible solution is either a central keratoprosthesis or a paralimbal scleral prosthesis. If the host cornea appears strong enough, a keratoprosthesis is implanted in the center of the corneal tissue. If the health of the host cornea appears compromised (i.e., the cornea is too thin or pseudocornea or anterior staphyloma is present), the same device is fixed to the nasal paralimbal sclera. We call this the "paralimbal scleral window," and it was first performed by Daljit Singh in 1982.

The keratoprosthesis that we use needs some explanation (Fig. 44.1).

The Singh–Worst Keratoprosthesis

The Singh–Worst keratoprosthesis is a one-piece polycarbonate device. The anterior surface of the device is convex, with a diameter of 6.0 mm, and has a flange. The flange merges into the shaft of the keratoprosthesis, which flares out posteriorly, thus forming a "neck" at the junction of the anterior surface and the body of the prosthesis. The end of the shaft has a diameter of 4.5 mm. The diameter at the level of the neck is 3.0 mm. The flange has eight equidistant holes near the margin. Four double-armed 80-μm stainless steel sutures are passed through these holes. This prosthesis is designed as a reverse cone that provides significantly better visibility for the fundus and excellent fixation, with less risk of extrusion (Fig. 44.2).

Fixation Concept of the Singh–Worst Keratoprosthesis

The basic idea behind the Singh–Worst design is to make the prosthesis absolutely immobile and minimize any micromovements between the prosthesis and the corneal or scleral bed. This is accomplished by using the dual-fixation principle. The prosthesis is fixed to the local host tissue around the waist as well to the sclera near the equator through the eight 80-μm steel sutures. The local fixation makes the opening watertight by tightening the host tissue around the neck of the keratoprosthesis, and the distant scleral fixation gives further stability, thus making it less vulnerable to extrusion. The stability of this prosthesis results from

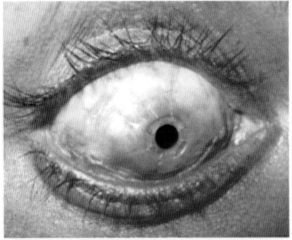

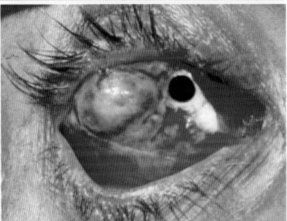

Figure 44.1. Central (**top**) and paralimbal (**bottom**) keratoprosthesis.

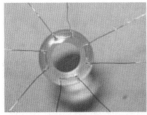 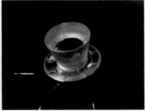

Figure 44.2. The Singh–Worst keratoprosthesis.

an equilibrium between the outward push of the intra-ocular pressure and the inward push by the distant sutures. The more the intra-ocular pressure tries to push the prosthesis out, the more snugly the anticonical shaft fits. Because of this dual-fixation principle, this is also known as the "champagne cork" keratoprosthesis. The fitting is like the cork in the champagne bottle, fitted tightly, with an extra harness of wires in place to secure it firmly. The tight but gentle local fixation keeps the host cornea from melting and prevents infectious agents from getting into the eye.

Indications for Surgery

All patients with corneal blindness, who are either outright unfit for keratoplasty or who have had multiple failed keratoplasty procedures, qualify for keratoprosthesis surgery. Patients with healthy corneal tissue are suitable for central keratoprosthesis, whereas a paralimbal scleral prosthesis is better suited for patients with thin corneal tissue or with pseudocornea. Common conditions include Stevens–Johnson syndrome, chemical burns, thermal burns, vascularized cornea following corneal ulcer, dry eye syndrome, and rheumatoid arthritis.

Preoperative Evaluation

The prognosis for keratoprosthesis procedures depends on the preoperative diagnosis. Keratoprostheses implanted in patients with ocular surface disorder (e.g., severe xerosis) tend to fare poorly as compared with patients with postcorneal ulcer scarring. Patients should be screened for good perception and projection of light, a normal posterior segment on B-scan ultrasonography, and normal intra-ocular pressure, checked digitally. If intraocular pressure is elevated, a filtration procedure is performed in the first stage to normalize pressure. A history of cataract surgery is important because in central keratoprosthesis, the crystalline lens or the intra-ocular lens must be removed. The patient and his or her family should be counseled regarding the possible outcome of the surgery and that prolonged postoperative care will be required.

Surgical Technique for Paralimbal Scleral Prosthesis

1. Perform conjunctival peritomy and sling the rectus muscles. Before proceeding further, estimate intra-ocular pressure by indenting the cornea with the tip of a needle holder. Evaluate corneal thickness and health. Identify any previously unnoticed or hidden scleral staphylomata (Fig. 44.3).

2. Spread the keratoprosthesis preloaded with sutures over the exposed eyeball. Do the preloading on a small eye drape so that steel sutures can be lifted one by one and anchored systematically in the sclera.

3. Implant the paralimbal window to the nasal paralimbal sclera and perform a free tenotomy of the medial rectus muscle to direct the prosthesis forward.

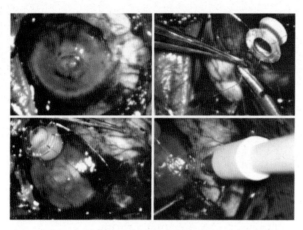

Figure 44.3. Peritomy is done, and 80-μm stainless steel sutures are passed through the sclera. A 2-mm marker is pressed on the site of paralimbal prosthesis.

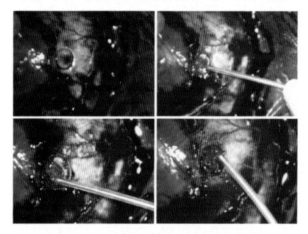

Figure 44.4. Fugo blade ablation of the marked area removes the sclera and starts ablation of the exposed ciliary body.

4. Pass all eight 80-μm steel sutures through the scleral tissue equidistant from each other, and keep the intended prosthesis implantation point at the center, at or near the equator of the globe, taking deep bites, with the sutures put in over half-sclera deep. Pass some sutures over the cornea as well. Once the scleral sutures are in place, push the keratoprosthesis aside slightly and use a 2.0-mm dermal biopsy trephine to make a mark on the paralimbal sclera.

5. Use the Fugo blade to slowly ablate the sclera and the underlying ciliary body, layer by layer until you reach the vitreous. This procedure is totally bloodless. In our case, earlier we used a trephine to make the initial opening (Fig. 44.4).

6. Make a full-thickness relaxing incision with the Fugo blade, parallel to the limbus in the opening

thus created (Fig. 44.5). (Traditionally this has been done with Castroviejo scissors.)

7. Also perform an anterior vitrectomy to reduce the chances of a retroprosthetic membrane. Use the Fugo blade to do a vitrectomy.

8. Pass a preplaced 80-μm steel suture across the relaxing incision.

9. Slip the posterior body of the keratoprosthesis through the opening and tighten the steel suture sufficiently to grip the prosthesis (Fig. 44.6). If need be, another suture may also be placed.

10. Once you have achieved local immobilization, pull the eight 80-μm sutures together and tie adjacent sutures together with square knots to avoid slippage. Form a total of four knots. The sutures should be just tight enough to give a slightly puffed appearance to the eyeball.

11. Inject fluid into the eyeball to make it just firm enough to keep the wound sealed and to buffer early postoperative intra-ocular pressure spikes.

12. Suture the conjunctiva back in place.

In patients with slightly weak corneal tissue or dry keratinized conjunctiva, a buccal mucosal graft is done around the keratoprosthesis. The graft will provide additional strength to the corneal tissue and an extra source of much-needed lubrication. Sometimes, if the anterior bulbar tissues are very weak to begin with, only a buccal mucosal transplant is done in the first stage, followed by keratoprosthesis surgery several weeks or months later.

When implanting a central keratoprosthesis, the basic technique remains the same except that the

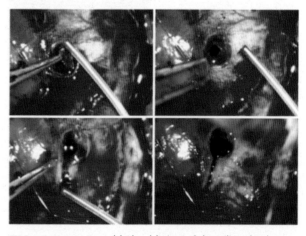

Figure 44.5. Fugo blade ablation of the ciliary body creates a hole in it. A linear relaxing incision is made in the decompressed soft eye.

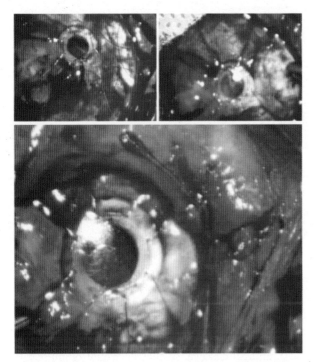

Figure 44.6. The keratoprosthesis is slipped inside. The relaxing incision is tied. The scleral sutures are tightened and tied. The conjunctiva is pulled back. The final image shows the condition of the eye at the end of the surgery.

opening is made in the center of the corneal tissue and the crystalline/cataractous lens must be removed before implanting the prosthesis.

Postoperative Management

Vision results after surgery are most surprising. Patients who undergo paralimbal scleral prosthesis surgery and have a good outcome can do nearly as well as the central-prosthesis group. They can walk around unaided and perform near-vision tasks with good dexterity. Vision does improve with the help of prescription glasses. In our series, most patients required glasses around +7.0 D spherical, which also works as a low-vision aid.

Postoperative Complications

Immediate Complications

It is not uncommon for acute glaucoma to develop in the early postoperative period, but it usually subsides in 1 to 2 weeks. The severity of postoperative inflammation varies from patient to patient. Any bleeding behind the prosthesis usually clears up in a few days.

Late Complications

Late complications after surgery can usually be handled successfully.

Glaucoma may continue perpetually after surgery in some patients. Intra-ocular pressure can only be tested digitally. The optic disc should be examined periodically whenever possible. These patients may need to continue on topical and oral antiglaucoma agents for a long time. If glaucoma is uncontrolled, transciliary filtration surgery can be performed to manage it.

Inflammatory and pigment deposits and thin retroprosthetic membrane can be cut using the yttrium–aluminum–garnet (YAG) laser; however, because of the length of the body of the device, a lot of pitting occurs. A thick retroprosthetic membrane has to be cut from the back using a 26-gauge needle. Thick vascularized membranes are cut with the Fugo blade. Most of the retroprosthetic membranes are inflammatory in nature. A course of antiinflammatory drugs usually clears them up.

Retinal detachment, if detected, can be treated by regular vitreoretinal procedures using a no-touch wide-angle viewing system.

The Singh–Worst prosthesis never extrudes completely because of the nature of its unique fixation. A loose local fixation can be reinforced with an 80-μm suture that regrips the prosthesis. In the 80-μm sutures loosen, the harness suture can be tightened by twisting the knot until it becomes tight again. If the harness suture becomes extremely loose, a new 80-μm suture can be used to stabilize it.

Endophthalmitis should be treated as with any normal patient.

Summary

Keratoprosthesis implantation surgery is a challenging surgery, in which no two eyes being operated on are the same. Keratoprosthesis presents wonderful opportunities for the prospect of restoring sight to corneal-blind individuals. The Fugo blade has contributed to this surgery by helping to make the surgery easier and safer.

Suggested Reading

Singh D. Keratoprosthesis. *Indian J Ophthalmol.* 1984;932: 405–407.

Singh I. Central and paracentral perforating keratoprosthesis— an experience of 200 cases. *Refract Corneal Surg.* 9:191–192.

Singh IR. Paralimbal scleral window. *An Inst Barraquer (Barc).* 2001;30:91–93.

45 Large Anterior Staphyloma DALJIT SINGH

Fungal, bacterial, or mixed corneal infections are common in poor countries. Corneal infections result from neglect of the infectious processes from the start and ineffectiveness of treatment once started. Partial or total anterior staphyloma are common; all that is left is to make the patient comfortable or to do some kind of surgery to improve their appearance. Sometimes an unusual situation calls for an innovative solution. As the following two cases illustrate, the Fugo blade can be included in surgery when tissue ablation or incision is involved.

CASE STUDIES

Case 1

The patient was a 30-year-old, very poor man in whom a large anterior staphyloma had developed after corneal ulceration 1 year before. The staphyloma jutted out between the lids and remained exposed day and night, causing great discomfort. Light perception was present and intra-ocular pressure (measured digitally) was very high. Bouts of pain left the patient incapacitated for hours. He and his family were on the verge of starvation because of his inability to work.

Many treatments were available to this patient. However, keratoplasty would be costly and beyond the patient's financial capability. And because donor corneas were unavailable, even free of charge, keratoplasty was out of the question. The patient insisted that I remove his disfigured, painful eye and outfit him with an artificial eye, so that he would be more presentable for hiring. We refused that course of treatment because the eye had light perception. Moreover, an artificial eyeball requires great care to maintain a healthy socket. We found a treatment that would reduce the patient's high intra-ocular pressure, contain the unsightly staphyloma, and offer a quick recovery so that he could return to work.

Surgical Technique

There was no anterior chamber and the patient's intra-ocular pressure was high. As a first step, intra-ocular pressure had to be reduced. Glaucoma surgery was performed by injecting visco-elastic material through a corneal pocket incision to separate the iris from the cornea. Iridectomy was done with the Fugo blade, and ab interno filtration followed. The patient was called back after 1 week for staphylectomy. The surgery was done as described below.

1. Check the intraocular pressure digitally. In our case, it appeared normal, but low pressure was required before we could proceed with the surgery.

2. Verify the filtration track by passing a curved cannula through the pocket incision in the cornea and the filtration track. In our case, the track appeared sufficient, but the flow of the injected fluid was sluggish.

3. Repeat ab interno filtration through the previously made corneal pocket incision. Test patency by injecting trypan blue into the anterior chamber.

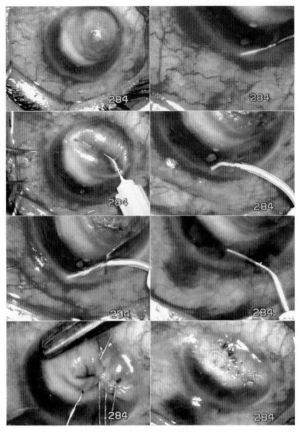

Figure 45.1. Subtotal anterior staphyloma (Case 1). Ab interno filtration is done through a corneal pocket incision. The edges of the staphyloma are infolded and joined together with 80-μm stainless steel sutures.

4. Judge the ocular pressure by pressing the staphyloma with a cannula. In our case, the eye appeared soft.

5. Infold the staphyloma with multiple 80-μm vanadium steel sutures. In our case, each suture picked somewhat healthier cornea beyond the staphyloma at one edge. This was then passed through the other edge across the staphyloma.

6. Begin suturing at one side and end on the opposite side. In our case, the soft eye allowed for infolding of the staphylomatous tissue with little resistance (Fig. 45.1).

Postoperative Management

Postoperatively, the patient was very comfortable and extremely satisfied. He returned to work 3 days after surgery. When the patient returned for follow-up 4 months later, the eye was quiet, there was no

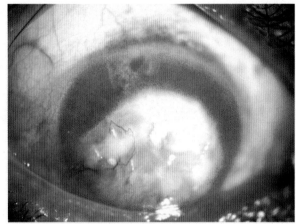

Figure 45.2. The appearance of the eye (Case 1) 4 months after surgery.

staphyloma, the sutures were in place, and his digital intra-ocular pressure appeared normal. He was able to see hand movements through the iridectomy at the 12 o'clock position. The sutures were in place and did not irritate the eye. The sutured tissues appeared to have fused the edges of the staphyloma (Fig. 45.2).

Case 2

The patient was a 23-year-old farm worker in whom an ocular deformity had developed in one eye after an injury and infection, resulting in loss of vision, 5 years previously. Because he could not close the eye while blinking and sleeping, he was bothered by the constant sensation of having a foreign body in his eye. He requested that I remove the eyeball and replace it with an artificial eye.

Examination showed a staphyloma extending from limbus to limbus; it looked like a cannonball. Digital tonometry appeared to be normal. The surgery was done as described below.

Surgical Technique

1. Make a horizontal incision with a 100-μm Fugo blade. In our case, it became apparent that the fibrovascular staphyloma tissue was very thick.

2. Deepen the limbus-to-limbus incision until the posterior surface of the pseudocornea is reached. In our case, the pseudocornea was more than 3 mm thick.

3. Both above and below the initial incision line, excise the pseudocornea using a forceps and a

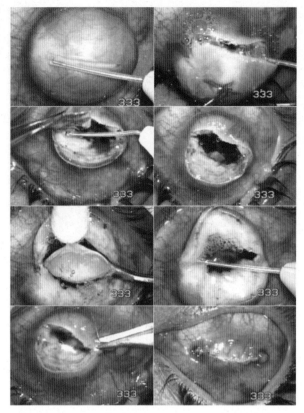

Figure 45.3. Total anterior staphyloma (Case 2) is incised, excised, and pared with the Fugo blade. The crystalline lens is removed. The edges of the cut staphyloma are sutured with 80-μm vanadium steel sutures.

Fugo blade at high power and high energy setting. There should be no bleeding.

4. Remove the crystalline lens. Remove the vitreous around it with a sponge.

5. Incise the deepest tissue in the staphyloma from the limbus before beginning the suturing.

6. Use multiple vanadium steel 80-μm sutures to close the gap resulting from the partial excision of the staphyloma (Figs. 45.3 and 45.4).

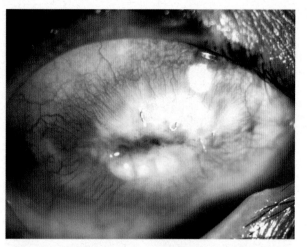

Figure 45.4. The operated eye (Case 2) 3 months after surgery. The eye is quiet and completely healed.

Postoperative Management

Two weeks after surgery, one loose irritating steel suture was removed. A thin gap in one area of the incision indicated that the wound was not closed, but a Seidel test was negative. Three months later, the site appeared the same as before and the eye was quiet.

Summary

The two cases described above demonstrate the utility of the Fugo blade in managing unusual cases in novel ways. These cases also show how minimally traumatic filtration surgery can be integrated with a primary surgical procedure.

Suggested Reading

Grieser EJ, Tuli SS, Chabi A, et al. Blueberry eye: acquired total anterior staphyloma after a fungal corneal ulcer. *Cornea.* 2009;28:231–232.

Part K
The Orbit

Dermoid of the Orbit DALJIT SINGH

The patient in this case presented with a huge orbital cyst that appeared at the upper lid. She also had severe hypotropia and ptosis. She was a poor man's daughter, and they could not afford to travel to seek help from an orbital or oculoplastic surgeon. We used the Fugo blade to excise the cyst.

TECHNIQUE

Anesthesia

Administer general anesthesia.

Surgical Technique

1. Make a skin incision over the most prominent part of the cyst. In this case, when the cyst was reached, I attempted to separate it from the surrounding tissues with a 100-μm capsulotomy tip. It quickly became apparent that it would be impossible to remove the cyst in toto without making a huge incision. I decided to drain the cyst before removing the cyst wall.

2. Make a 1-cm incision in the thick cyst wall. In this case, I removed a large amount of cheesy material and hair by applying pressure to the outside of the eye and scooping material from inside.

3. I attempted to separate the wall of the empty cyst with the same ablation tip but stopped because the tip was very soft and flexible, it was taking far too long, and it could not be done without magnified vision.

4. Excise the anterior part of the wall that has been separated from the surrounding tissues. In this case, I was able to remove the rest of the contents of the cyst through a large hole.

5. Perform all further dissection, separation, and cutting with a blunt scissors aided by an artery forceps. Minor bleeding may be controlled by applying pressure. Remove the cyst completely, leaving the bed of the cyst very smooth.

6. Close the incision line in two layers, the orbicularis and the skin. Use 80-μm vanadium steel sutures. In this case, recovery was uneventful (Fig. 46.1).

46

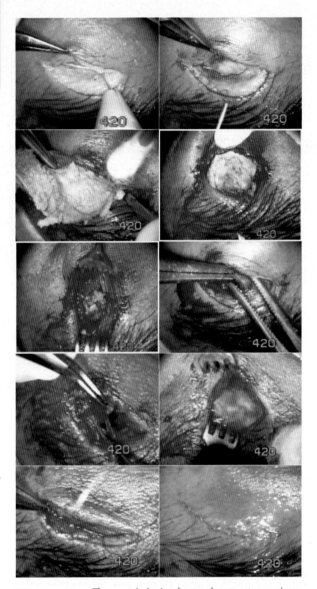

Figure 46.1. The cyst is incised over the most prominent projection and separated from the surrounding tissues with a 100-μm Fugo blade tip. A 1-cm incision is made in the cyst, and a large amount of cheesy material and hair is expressed. The visible cyst wall is excised to expose and remove more contents. The emptied cyst is held with artery forceps, and further isolation and excision of the wall is done with a scissors. The smooth bed of the cyst is visible. The incision is closed in two layers with 80-μm steel sutures.

Summary

This surgery was a unique and exhilarating experience for me because I had never ventured so far into the orbit. Subsequently, I discovered that blunt dissection could be done bloodlessly using a 600-μm Fugo blade tip. If I were to encounter a similar case tomorrow, I would alter the surgical technique slightly as follows.

1. Incise the skin with 100-μm tip and reach the cyst.
2. Use scissors to dissect the cyst away from the orbital contents.
3. Incise the cyst wall and drain or remove the contents of the cyst.
4. Close the incised cyst with 80-μm steel sutures.
5. Grasp the cyst with an artery forceps and pull it out from every direction. Continue separating the cyst from the surrounding tissues with a 600-μm Fugo blade until all of the cyst is removed in one piece.

Suggested Reading

Winn CW. Broad applications seen for plasma blade. *Ocular Surg News Asia Pacific Ed*. 2001;19:45–46.

Part L
The Globe

Evisceration DALJIT SINGH

E visceration is the removal of the contents of the globe while leaving the sclera and extra-ocular muscles intact. Evisceration is usually indicated in endophthalmitis that does not respond to medication or for cosmetic improvement of a blind eye.

The patient is informed that it is impossible to achieve or retain any vision with this procedure and that removal of the eye is essential to resolve the inflammation or unsightliness of the eye. The patient is also counseled regarding the form of cosmetic improvement to be expected, with or without inserting an implant within the empty scleral shell, either at surgery or at some future point.

No case of sympathetic ophthalmia after evisceration has been reported. If the slightest chance of saving some useful sight in trauma cases exists, the eye should not undergo evisceration.

The primary challenge in operating on soft infected eyes is making a clean incision on a soft cornea or limbus. A secondary consideration is the possibility of spreading infection through the channels by cutting manually with a knife or scissors. Both these challenges can be overcome by making incisions with a Fugo blade.

Surgical Technique

1. Use a 100-μm Fugo blade tip set at medium power and high energy to incise the cornea near the limbus. Move the activated tip along the desired incision line inside the limbus and continue to make a gutter in the cornea. Because the cornea is usually thick in these cases, it takes two or three passes to go through and reach inside the eye. Make the incision in such a way that no infected tissue is kept at the incision margin. If an infective process is invading the sclera, make the incision proximally so as to pass through healthy sclera.

    The sharpest cutting knives, including diamond knives, often cannot make a clean-cut incision because they can work only in the presence of tissue resistance. They are not suitable for use in infected, soft eyes. But the Fugo blade cuts either a soft eye or a hard eye with equal facility.

2. Cut the uveolenticular mass. Lift the incised corneal tissue to reveal the inflammatory mass, lens, vitreous, and uveal tissues, inextricably mixed. In the central area, pull and excise this mass with the Fugo blade.

3. Pull the ciliary body away from the sclera and insert a spatula in the suprachoroidal space, thus separating the sclera from the uveal–retinal tissue. Move the spatula around in every direction and as deep into the sclera as possible. Remove the entire mass with several scrapes of the spatula (Fig. 47.1). My colleagues and I do not use evisceration spoons because they cause excessive trauma to the internal surface of the sclera. Surgical trauma should be minimized in infected cases.

4. Rinse the empty scleral cavity with povidine–iodine.

Any additional surgical steps are determined by several factors, such as the age of the patient, original cause of the loss of the eye, and any cosmetic treatment planned.

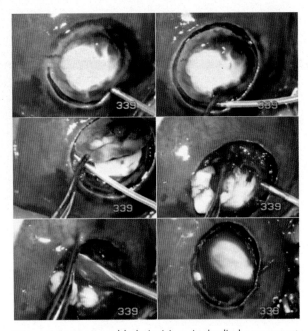

Figure 47.1. Fugo blade incisions in the limbus area cut the cornea to full depth. The uveovitreolenticular mass is excised. A spatula is introduced in the suprachoroidal space to remove the contents. The scleral cavity is cleared of tissue.

Summary

The Fugo blade's capacity to cut successfully in situations in which no tissue resistance is present has stimulated interest in harvesting sclerocorneal buttons from cadaver eyes, which are transferred directly to preservative medium bottles.

Suggested Reading

Albert DM, Diaz-Rohena R. A historical review of sympathetic ophthalmia and its epidemiology. *Surv Ophthalmol.* 1989;34:1–14.

Hemophthalmos SEEMA K. SINGH

What follows is a description of the surgical management of a case of hemophthalmos using the Fugo blade in surgical procedures that were unimaginable only a few years ago.

The patient in this case was an 11-year-old child who had already undergone extracapsular cataract extraction and iris claw lens implantation for a traumatic cataract 6 years previously. The patient presented 6 days after severe blunt trauma that resulted in hemophthalmos. The child was in severe pain and the intra-ocular pressure was very high. The lids were swollen. We did not expect light to penetrate through so much dark blood, but the patient did have very limited light perception.

There was blood everywhere in the eye. A B-scan revealed that both the vitreous and the anterior chamber were full of blood. The anterior chamber showed a blackball hemorrhage over three quarters of the eye and dark red blood over the rest of the eye (Fig. 48.1). Ultrasound B-mode did not show a posterior chamber, as if this cavity too had been squeezed by the blood.

To treat this patient successfully, the anterior chamber would have to be cleared and the intra-ocular pressure should be brought under control. My colleagues and

I planned to evaluate the patient's progress and refer her to a vitreoretinal surgeon if the vitreous did not clear up spontaneously within a reasonable period.

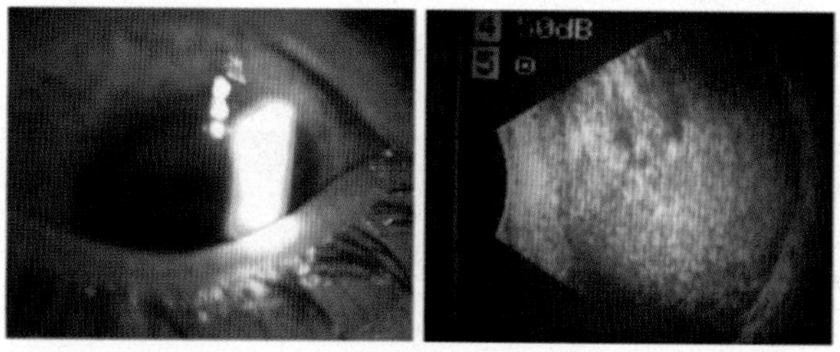

From a surgical standpoint, mere paracentesis was impossible because the angle structures would be thoroughly clogged with blood. Starting the treatment from the vitreous side would have been a blind procedure unless an endoscopic device was available with vitrectomy.

We reasoned that tapping into the posterior chamber would yield some results because aqueous fluid could not flow freely and was collecting in the posterior chamber.

TECHNIQUE

Anesthesia

Perform the operation under general anesthesia.

Surgical Technique

In our case, the eye was observed to be highly congested. Touching on the cornea indicated that the intra-ocular pressure was very high.

1. Perform transconjunctival transciliary filtration in the upper outer quadrant.

2. In our case, clear aqueous was observed flowing from the posterior chamber.

3. We irrigated the posterior chamber with saline and rinsed out a small quantity of clotted blood (Fig. 48.2).

Figure 48.1. Initial presentation of the eye shows a blackball hemorrhage in the anterior chamber. A B-scan shows that the vitreous is full of blood.

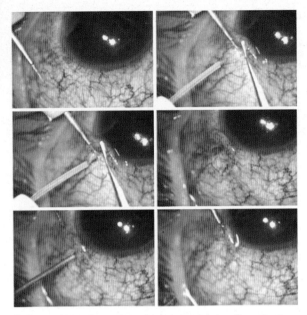

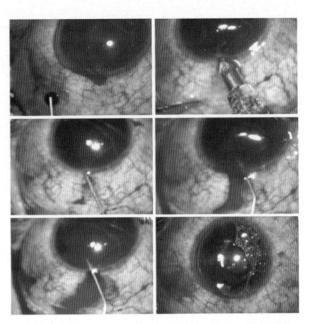

Figure 48.2. Blackball hemorrhage. The conjunctiva is slid toward the limbus and held down about 1 mm behind the surgical limbus. An activated 300-μm Fugo blade tip is passed along the blunt diamond conjunctival retractor that holds down the conjunctiva, through the conjunctiva, through the sclera and the ciliary body, and into the posterior chamber. Pigment and a minimal amount of blood flows out along with the aqueous. The posterior chamber is rinsed with saline to ensure that no blood remains in the cavity.

Figure 48.3. Trypan blue dropped on the conjunctival open wound confirms continued fluid drainage. The anterior chamber is opened at the 12 o'clock position. The anterior chamber is repeatedly washed with urokinase 1:10,000. Finally, a large air bubble is placed in the anterior chamber.

4. Make a stab incision at the 12 o'clock position. Repeatedly irrigate the anterior chamber with urokinase solution at 10,000 units per milliliter. Within 15 minutes, the anterior chamber in our case appeared to be reasonably clear of blood (Fig. 48.3).

5. Place a large air bubble in the anterior chamber.

Postoperative Management

Twenty-four hours after surgery, the eye was quiet. The anterior chamber showed a medium-sized air bubble. Slightly dark red blood occupied three quarters of the anterior chamber and movement of the air bubble indicated that the blood was fluid (Fig. 48.4).

Two days later the anterior chamber was cleared with repeated saline irrigation and aspiration.

On the fourth day after surgery, the anterior chamber was clear and the iris claw lens was visible (Fig. 48.5). There was no congestion in the eye, and the patient had light projection in all directions. A well-formed bleb appeared to be formed from clear

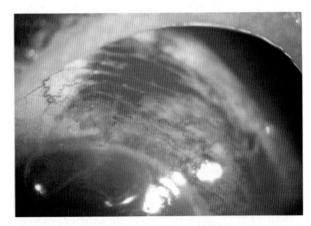

Figure 48.4. One day after surgery. Filtration is restored; some blood has entered the lymphatics. A large air bubble is present in the anterior chamber.

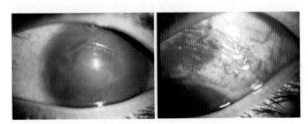

Figure 48.5. Four days after surgery. The anterior chamber is almost clear. The conjunctiva apart from the surgical site shows no congestion. The bleb is well formed.

48

aqueous. Blood filled many lymphatic vessels running parallel to the limbus.

Summary

At this point it is still too early to determine this patient's prospects for vision recovery. But this case successfully proves that it is possible to drain the posterior chamber of a badly damaged eye that has high intra-ocular pressure. The prospect affords both patient and surgeon some breathing room and the confidence to plan subsequent treatment to restore sight.

Suggested Reading

Kellan R, Fugo RJ. Device increases safety, efficiency of cataract surgery. *Ophthalmol Times*. 2000;25:7–9.

Roy FH. Course of Fugo blade is enlightening, surgeon says. *Ocular Surg News*. 2001;19:35–38.

Section III
Nonophthalmic Applications of the Fugo Blade

The Fugo Blade in General Surgery: Experimental Work*

G. RUSSELL REISS

The Fugo blade is a novel electrosurgical device that was designed for ophthalmologic use. Its principles of operation are based on the applied photon bath theory of plasma ablation. Using carbon-based tissue in its path as a fuel source to generate a "cool" cloud of high-intensity plasma energy, the Fugo blade can create a pristine incision in the various tissues of the eye while simultaneously achieving hemostasis in highly vascular fields. At this time, a commercial plasma-based cutting device such as the Fugo blade does not exist for extra-ocular use. The current state of the art in general surgery is the handheld electrocautery, otherwise known as the Bovie. Unfortunately, the Bovie lacks thermal efficiency, often rendering tissues charred and burned as the surrounding tissues at the point of contact act as a heat sink for its extreme high-temperature cutting and coagulation. Although several attempts have been made to harness the laserlike energy deployed by the Fugo blade and apply it for wide application in general surgical procedures, these devices suffer from many limitations and risks. Most notably, surgical lasers based on energy similar to plasma are expensive, bulky, and fraught with dangerous complications such as past pointing and the potential to blind operative staff inadvertently.

Based on the Fugo blade's reported mechanism of operation we hypothesized that the Fugo blade M100 unit could be used for surgical incision of nonocular tissues. To test this hypothesis, we performed several nonocular operations on both rodent and nonrodent species.

Equipment

Workstation

Our standard surgical workstation for small animals consists of a stainless steel surgical cart specially designed for small animal surgery. On this cart, we have an anesthesia machine and heated induction chamber, which can deliver oxygen, isoflurane volatile anesthetic, or a mixture of the two. Other components of the operative theater include a small animal respirator for experiments requiring mechanical ventilation, a warming unit for the operating stage, a high-intensity fiber-optic light source, an operating microscope and various microsurgical instruments. The M100 unit fits nicely on the workstation, with the foot pedal easily positioned under the surgical stool and the handpiece placed on the operative field, making it accessible for use throughout the entire procedure (Fig. 49.1).

*This manuscript is the result of work supported with resources from and the use of facilities at the George E. Wahlen VA Medical Center and by a grant from the Western Institute for Biomedical Research.

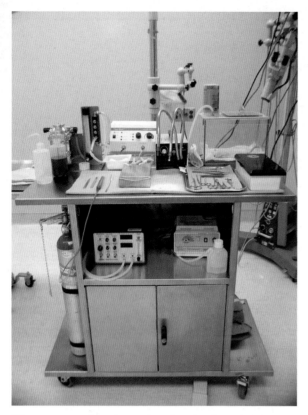

Figure 49.1. Experimental workstation featuring the Fugo blade M100 unit.

Fugo Blade M100 Unit

Because the surgical fields in operations pertaining to the eye are quite small and confined, the original Fugo blade M100 unit developed for ophthalmology uses very low power (3 W). Our initial benchtop experiments indicated that this standard M100 unit was underpowered for small animal surgery in nonocular tissues. We therefore had MediSurg, Ltd. modify the Fugo blade circuitry to allow a modest increase in power output without changing the characteristics of the plasma profile generated from the device. This minor modification proved to be sufficient for initial proof-of-concept studies.

Tips

The Fugo blade's traditional cutting tips are quite fine and are available in right-angled 100-μm and straight 400-μm filaments. We found that these standard tips were quite delicate even for small animal surgery, especially the 100-μm version. We therefore elected not to use the 100-μm filament for macro tissue cutting, such as skin incisions, and evaluated its use for only the most delicate of procedures. We

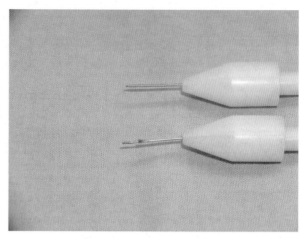

Figure 49.2. Modified 400-μm Fugo blade tip.

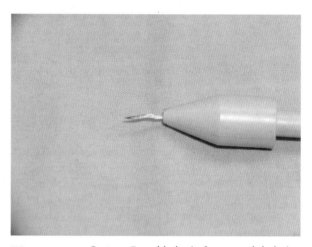

Figure 49.3. Custom Fugo blade tip for nonophthalmic surgery.

modified the straight 400-μm tip by excising a small portion of the insulating sheath approximately 4 mm back from the terminal end (Fig. 49.2). In addition, we also had MediSurg, Ltd. design a specialized, more durable tip for cutting thicker tissues, such as skin and muscle (Fig. 49.3). The result of these modifications allowed the surgeon to quickly move about the surgical field, which was not afforded with the standard tips.

Materials and Methods

Animals

Prior to investigation we obtained approval from the George E. Wahlen VA Institutional Animal Care and Use Committee for all procedures. We purchased

49

specific pathogen-free animals from established vendors known to the VA.

Initial Benchtop Testing

Before embarking on survival surgeries, benchtop cutting was performed and evaluated on euthanized animals to calibrate the level of power needed for various tissues in rats and rabbits. In these nonsurvival surgeries, complete autopsy and vivisection was performed using various levels of cut power and cut intensity. These power and intensity adjustments were easily performed by manipulating the two large dials on the front of the M100 unit.

Rodent Studies

After completing a series of benchtop evaluations, we performed multiple survival procedures on animals that would otherwise have undergone surgery using scalpels, scissors, and standard monopolar electrocautery. These procedures included both laparotomies with abdominal exploration and thoracotomies, including mediastinal procedures on the heart. In two separate experimental groups, six 250-g, female, Sprague Dawley rats were operated on. In the first set of animals, we performed survival abdominal surgery by performing a paramedian laparotomy. Skin incision was performed using the Fugo blade tip made specifically for our lab (Fig. 49.4). Once through the skin, this tip was exchanged for the modified 400-μm tip to continue further dissection (Fig. 49.5). Although a full-thickness incision could have been performed in one fell swoop, we elected to carefully dissect and divide the abdominal wall in layers following the natural planes of dissection.

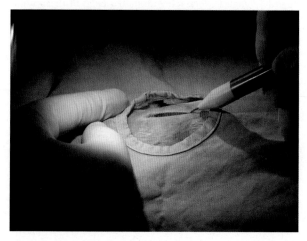

Figure 49.4. Skin incision using a custom Fugo blade tip.

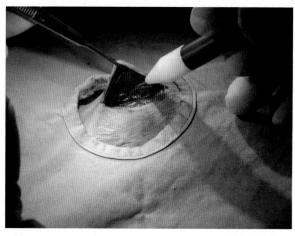

Figure 49.5. Tissue dissection using a modified 400-μm Fugo blade tip.

In the second group of rodents, a left anterolateral thoracotomy was performed using a midline, chest skin incision. Again, after using the customized tip for the skin, the rest of the operation was performed with the modified straight 400-μm tip. With this operation, it is imperative to have complete control over the depth and intensity of the energy produced at the cutting interface, as the small rodent lungs and pleura are extremely delicate and highly susceptible to injury as one enters the left chest. Normally, the left chest would be entered only with cold-instrument, blunt dissection, as the risk of puncturing the visceral pleura on the lung surface is too great. However, the 400-μm tip set on high cut power with a low-to-moderate cut intensity setting was used to enter the thoracic cage for all procedures. In both groups of animals, incisions were closed in layers using running absorbable suture. Animals were allowed to recover in a dedicated, warm postoperative cage and then returned to the animal facility for routine postoperative care and husbandry.

Nonrodent Studies

Our lab also routinely performs thoracotomies in New Zealand white rabbits for an established coronary ligation model. After completion of rodent studies with the Fugo blade, we evaluated the M100 unit for its cutting and dissection properties in six of this much larger animal. Again, using the customized tip for skin incision, a left lateral thoracotomy was performed through a left anterior lateral chest-wall incision. The underlying latissimus dorsi and serratus anterior muscles were dissected and divided in layers and the thoracic cage was entered through the seventh intercostal space using the modified, 400-μm straight tip.

Once the interthoracic procedure was complete, the chest cage and chest wall muscles and the skin were closed in layers using running absorbable sutures. Animals were allowed to recover in a dedicated, warm postoperative cage and then returned to the animal facility for routine postoperative care and husbandry.

Results

In all animal experiments the Fugo blade provided clean, precise, cutting and tissue ablation. All animals, both rodent and nonrodent, survived the operations and made a complete recovery. At 2 weeks, after surgery all animals were killed and underwent autopsy. The skin incisions were excised and evaluated for tissue integrity and completeness of wound healing. There was excellent tissue recovery and integrity at 14 days in all animals with histology revealing only moderate inflammatory response in the areas of suture placement. In the rodent experiments, which are notably less sanguinous than larger animals, bleeding control was excellent, with virtually no hemorrhage noted or attributable to the Fugo blade. With regard to tissue incision, the Fugo blade was much superior to cold-instrument, blunt dissection, as it allowed exacting control over division of tissue planes without tearing. Upon entering the chest cavity proper, the fine 400-μm tip with the M100 set on the lower cut intensity setting allowed reproducible surgical entrance to the thorax without risk of injury to the underlying lung. In the rabbit experiments, the M100 unit performed very well for cutting and ablation but was unable to provide the same level of complete hemostasis as seen with the rodents. This was particularly true when dividing the larger diameter (>1 mm) crossing vessels and muscle perforators. However, this limitation did not pose any risk or threat to the animals or impede the success of the operations, as these vessels are easily controlled with the crush-clamp technique using a fine hemostat.

Summary

Not since the introduction of the Bovie by Dr. Harvey Cushing in 1926, has there been a widely applicable, safe, and efficient advance in electrosurgical technology such as the Fugo blade. As clearly demonstrated in the above preliminary experiments, the Fugo Blade is a scalable technology that can be used for surgical cutting and ablation in virtually any tissue and in any cavity of the body. The less-than-complete hemostasis seen in the rabbit model can be attributed to our use of a slightly modified M100 unit that was originally designed for the much smaller ocular space and for much finer and more delicate surgery. Had MediSurg, Ltd. made available a larger more powerful unit, we feel strongly that this larger vessel control would not have been an issue. In spite of this minor limitation, the "turbocharged" version of the M100 Fugo blade allowed precision cutting and ablation that is not otherwise available to the general or thoracic surgeon at this time. Probably the most promising aspect of the Fugo blade is found in its unique ability to cut effortlessly through tissues while minimizing the surrounding thermal injury. By design, the Fugo blade cuts only in the most focused part of the plasma cloud that is generated mere micrometers from the activated tip surface. This is quite a contrast from standard electrosurgical units that are based on diathermy, and trade off what can sometimes be extensive thermal injury for cutting and hemostasis. In summary, these proof-of-concept small animal studies demonstrate that the Fugo blade can be successfully scaled for use in nonocular applications in general and thoracic surgery.

Suggested Reading

Fugo RJ, Singh D, Fine IH. Automated Fugo blade capsulotomy: a new technique and a new instrument. *Eyeworld*. 2002;7:49–54.

Massarweh NN, Cosgriff N, Slakey DP. Electrosurgery: history, principles, and current and future uses. *J Am Coll Surg*. 2006;202:520–530.

The Fugo Blade in Treatment of the Ear, Nose, and Throat

AMRIK SINGH

T echnologic progress forever changes how things are perceived and accomplished. The ear, nose, and throat (ENT) field is quite different now from what it was just a few years ago. Over the course of my 40 years of ENT practice, I gained extensive experience with treatment methods such as suction diathermy, cryosurgery, radiocautery, and the use of both the carbon dioxide laser and the potassium titanyl phosphate (KTP) laser. Although purportedly the most modern and cutting-edge techniques, carbon dioxide and KTP lasers come with their own set of problems.

In 2002, I heard about the characteristics of Fugo blade ablation from the ophthalmology department at my institution. I began to incorporate the Fugo blade into my ENT surgeries. Experience with the Fugo blade has shown that it has none of the disadvantages of standard ENT techniques and in fact offers many advantages.

The Fugo blade is a simple and safe tool to use and is easy to maintain. No special precautions must be taken, nor have my colleagues and I encountered any specific complications related to the device, either during surgery or postoperatively. By virtue of the Fugo blade's ablation and penetration properties, tissue definition is very good. The heat produced is more localized, so collateral tissue damage is negligible. The Fugo blade has proved to be advantageous over existing forms of treatment (Table 50.1). Additional advantages

include its reliability and relatively low cost, compact dimensions, and lightweight portability. Many procedures that once involved overnight or longer stays at a hospital are now treated in an outpatient setting using the Fugo blade.

To date, I have treated a variety of ENT conditions and performed a range of surgical techniques using the Fugo blade with great success (Table 50.2). Several illustrative examples are described below.

The Larynx

Use of the Fugo blade (rather than a laser, with its accompanying fumes) allows the surgeon to effectively concentrate on the laryngeal structures and treat them with minimal tissue excision and minimal rupture of the superficial lamina propria.

Vocal Nodules

Vocal nodules appear on the free edge of the vocal cord at the junction of its anterior one third and posterior two thirds, the location of maximum cord vibration and hence subject to maximum trauma. Nodules can range in size from that of a pinhead to a small pea. Nodules develop as a result of vocal trauma, for example, when a person speaks in unnaturally low tones for prolonged periods or at high intensities. Vocal nodules

Table 50.1. Comparison of Conventional Surgical Methods with the Fugo Blade

Disadvantages of Carbon Dioxide Laser and KTP Laser	Advantages of the Fugo Blade
Staff training required. Every staff member in the operating room must don special protective eyewear.	Minimal training required; no special preparation needed before or during surgery
Difficult and prolonged learning curve for proper handling	Easy to handle
Imprecise and inaccurate skin and soft-tissue dissection	Precise and accurate skin and soft-tissue dissection
Poor tissue definition	Better tissue definition
Palpable collateral tissue damage	No collateral tissue damage
Thermal damage to some tissues (e.g., laryngeal and tracheal cartilage) results in fibrosed tissue.	Laryngeal and tracheal cartilage tissues are easy to divide with minimal damage.
Severe postoperative tissue reaction and edema	Minimal bleeding; almost no bleeding from capillaries
Slow re-epithelialization	No or minimal postoperative pain and tissue reaction or edema
Extensive recovery period	Faster re-epithelization ensures faster healing and recovery.
	Short recovery period
	Better patient compliance with postoperative care and follow-up

Table 50.2. ENT Conditions Treated and Procedures Performed Successfully Using the Fugo Blade

Pathology/Condition	Surgical Procedures
Branchial sinus	Arytenoidectomy
Granuloma of the vocal process	Branchial cyst excision
Keloids (ear lobule, chest wall, upper arm)	Division of tongue tie
Laryngeal stenosis	Parotidectomy
Multiple juvenile laryngeal papillomas	Tonsillectomy
Nasolabial cyst	Uvulopalatopharyngoplasty
Pharyngeal stenosis	
Reinke's edema	
Septal papilloma	
Tracheal stenosis	
Tracheal stomal papilloma	
Ventricular cyst	
Vocal nodule	
Vocal polyp	

mostly affect teachers, singers, vendors, or actors and can also be seen in school-age children and adolescents. Patients with vocal nodules report hoarseness, vocal fatigue, and pain in the throat on prolonged phonation.

Early cases of vocal nodules can be treated conservatively by educating the patient about proper use of the voice. Surgery is required for large or long-standing nodules in adults.

Surgical Technique: Microlaryngeal Surgery with the Fugo Blade

1. Inspect and photograph the lesion to be treated (Fig. 50.1).
2. Ablate the nodule with the laryngeal probe of the Fugo blade (Fig. 50.2). The blade delivers

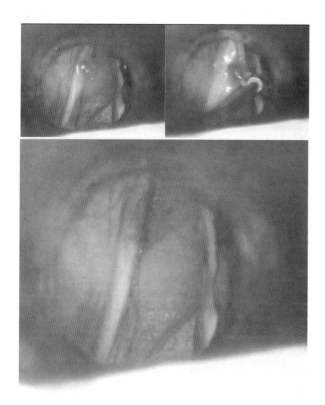

Figure 50.1. Vocal nodule before, during, and after surgery with the Fugo blade.

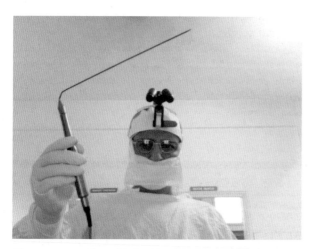

Figure 50.2. Fugo blade microlaryngeal probe.

plasma energy at the tip with outstanding precision and without clinically visible collateral damage. Even the surrounding normal epithelium is unaffected.

3. It takes only 5 to 7 minutes to very gradually remove the nodule or polyp.

4. To prevent recurrence of the nodule, penetrate the subepithelial space to a depth of 0.5 mm.

Postoperative Management

Postoperatively the vocal cord looks slightly swollen but heals and returns to normal within 2 weeks. Postoperative pain is nonexistent, and the patient is discharged the same day. If a laser were used for the same purpose, the recovery period would be much longer. The nodule has not recurred in any of the 11 cases I have treated with the Fugo blade.

Multiple Juvenile Laryngeal Papillomas

Juvenile-onset laryngeal papillomas are the most common cause of laryngeal tumors in children. They are caused by virally induced epithelial proliferation (human papillomavirus types 6 and 11). They tend to disappear after puberty, which demonstrates hormonal involvement to some extent. Papillomas appear as glistening, fleshy, wartlike, white irregular growths that are sessile (occasionally pedunculated), friable, and bleed easily (Fig. 50.3). They are benign and are

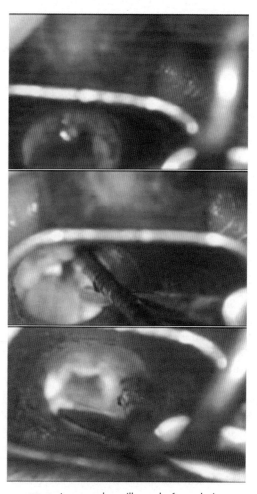

Figure 50.3. Laryngeal papilloma before, during, and after surgery with the Fugo blade.

50

seen mostly on the true and false vocal cords and the epiglottis. If they are allowed to advance, however, known complications include spreading to other sites in the larynx and tracheobronchial tree and to the nasopharynx and nasal vestibule, respiratory obstruction, and, rarely, malignant degeneration.

Patients usually present with chronic hoarseness and inspiratory dyspnea with stridor, which starts developing as the lesion advances. However, the condition does not necessarily present insidiously, and respiratory difficulty maybe its first manifestation. Diagnosis can easily be made with a pediatric fiberoptic nasopharyngoscope, which allows easy visualization of the larynx.

Laryngeal papillomas are undoubtedly one of the most challenging benign conditions facing the laryngologist, especially because of their propensity to recur. Many different methods, including conventional surgery; laser surgery; medical therapy with indole-3-carbinol, α-interferons, and acyclovir; and even photodynamic therapy have been used to treat patients with laryngeal papillomas, yet the multitude of methods seems to reflect the inability of a single individual method to control the disease.

The Fugo blade has been singularly helpful in treating this condition. It is very easy to ablate the papillomas in depth without damaging the submucosa. Tissue definition is good and precise dissection is possible. Healing takes place within a week and without scarring. Postoperative edema is minimal, and voice quality returns to near normal in virtually all patients. With lasers, 10 to 15 treatment sessions are necessary just to control the condition. With the Fugo blade however, 3 to 5 treatments are enough to control and even eradicate the disease. I have successfully treated 4 cases of juvenile laryngeal papillomas using the Fugo blade.

Laryngeal Cyst/Anterior Saccular Cyst

In the anterior ventricle of the larynx lies the sacculus laryngis, also known as the laryngeal saccule. This process contains numerous mucous glands, and its role is to express secretions to lubricate the vocal fold. Obstruction of the saccule causes secretion retention and saccule distention, which presents as a cyst in the laryngeal ventricle. Because there is no connection with the intralaryngeal lumen, it is called a "saccular cyst." It generally presents in the anterior part of the ventricle or posteriorly into the false vocal cord of the epiglottic fold. Patients generally present with a history of hoarseness. I have treated two such cases with the Fugo blade.

Surgery is done under general anesthesia. The standard method is marsupialization, which is an insufficient

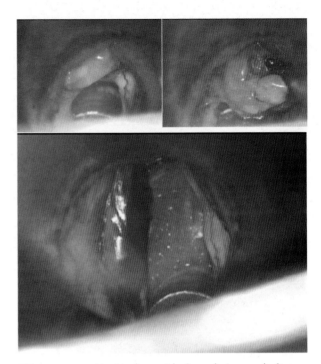

Figure 50.4. Ventricular cyst before, during, and after surgery with the Fugo blade.

treatment, because the cyst recurs in many patients. The effective treatment is complete excision of the cyst (Fig. 50.4). A recurrence requires a more extensive external approach.

Complete dissection of the laryngeal cyst is easy with the Fugo blade. Bleeding is negligible. The Fugo blade easily reaches the required depth for dissection, with clinically little collateral damage. Re-epithelization is rapid.

The Trachea

The use of Fugo blade to treat conditions of the trachea is illustrated with a few examples.

Tracheal Stomal Papillomas

When the Fugo blade is used to excise tracheal stomal papillomas, burning and charring of the tissue is remarkably absent (Fig. 50.5).

Tracheal Stenosis

Submucosal dissection of fibrous tissue using the plasma knife has made it possible to achieve the desired lumen size with the least amount of damage to the mucosa (Fig. 50.6).

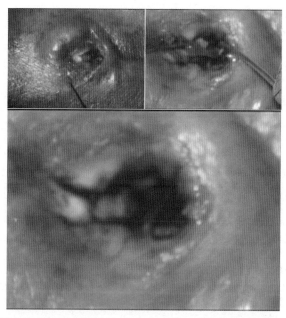

Figure 50.5. Tracheal stomal papilloma before, during, and after surgery with the Fugo blade.

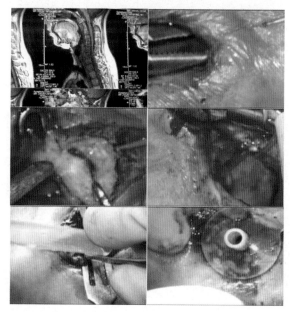

Figure 50.6. Computed tomographic scan showing the extent of tracheal stenosis. The surgical photographs show incision of the skin, exposure and cutting of the cricoid and tracheal cartilages with the Fugo blade, and dissection and excision of the fibrous tissue.

Oral Cavity and Oropharynx

Tonsillectomy

My colleagues and I first performed a tonsillectomy with a Fugo blade on a 40-year-old woman with tonsillitis. Since then, we have done many more tonsillectomies on

both adults and children and in some cases, on patients with large tonsils that interfered with the patient's swallowing and breathing, sometimes severely enough to cause sleep apnea.

Surgical Technique: Tonsillectomy

1. Make an incision with the Fugo blade only in the mucous membrane.

2. Separate the superior pole from the bed by separating the fibrous bands by just touching the activated Fugo blade tip to the tissue.

3. Cut the mucosa of the posterior pillar with the Fugo blade. The incision should be deep enough to reach the surgical capsule of the tonsil.

4. Use the Fugo blade to separate the tonsil and its capsule from the surrounding peritonsillar tissue.

5. Gripping the tonsil by its upper pole, continue to draw the tonsil toward the midline and continue the dissection with the Fugo blade to reach the lower pole. At this point, the firm fibrous fold is very easy to divide using the Fugo blade without much bleeding. It is very easy to dissect the tonsil completely (Fig. 50.7). However, it is important to note that the cutting power of the Fugo blade is slow, and as a result it does take longer to remove the tonsils.

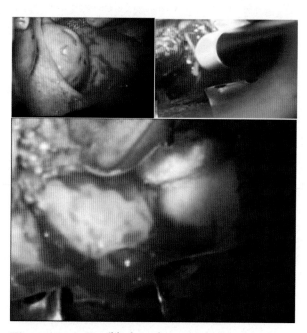

Figure 50.7. Tonsil before, during, and after surgery with the Fugo blade. The tonsillar bed is clean and is devoid of charring or tissue damage.

50

6. Minor bleeding is controlled quickly and effectively with the Fugo blade tip Occasionally, you may need to suture the paratonsillar vein with a silk thread.

Postoperative Management

Postoperatively less facial edema, inflammation, and slough formation is seen than with conventional dissection methods. Sloughing will disappear in about 10 to 12 days. Almost no tissue reaction occurs, and scarring of the tonsillar bed is minimal. Compared with micro-electrocautery tonsillectomy and laser tonsillectomy, the Fugo blade's thermal collateral damage is negligible, hence postoperative pain, slough formation, and complications such as hemorrhage and tissue fibrosis are significantly reduced. Patients treated with the Fugo blade return to their normal diet sooner than those who undergo blunt-dissection tonsillectomy.

Superficial Parotidectomy

As the first steps in superficial parotidectomy, it is very easy to dissect and raise a skin flap with the Fugo blade. Tissue dissection is precise, bleeding is minimal, and no collateral tissue damage occurs. A standard parotidectomy skin incision is shown in Figure 50.8.

TECHNIQUE

Anesthesia

Administer general anesthesia.

Surgical Technique: Superficial Parotidectomy

1. Make a standard parotidectomy skin incision (Fig. 50.8).
2. Deepen the incision below the mandible through the platysma down to the level of (but not into) the deep cervical fascia.
3. Using the Fugo blade, raise the skin and subcutaneous tissue flap anteriorly and the platysma inferiorly. Use silk sutures to hold the flaps. Hemostasis is effectively obtained with the plasma knife itself.

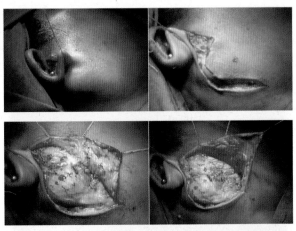
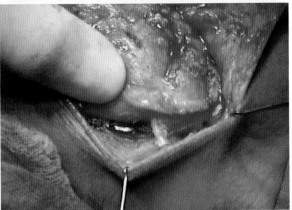
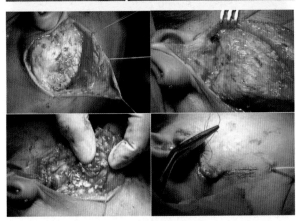

Figure 50.8. Superficial parotidectomy with the Fugo blade. The skin flap is raised, the greater auricular nerve is divided, the parotid gland is separated from the surrounding structures, and the facial nerve is exposed and identified. The tumor tissue is excised with the Fugo blade, preserving the facial nerve and its branches.

4. The greater auricular nerve lies on the deep cervical fascia investing the sternomastoid muscle. Separate the anterior border of the sternomastoid muscle using the Fugo blade from the posterior border of the parotid gland. Divide the greater

auricular nerve at the point where it crosses onto the parotid gland.

5. Further up, separate the gland from the mastoid process and the cartilaginous external meatus under the microscope.

6. Now deepen the sulcus by sharp dissection to expose the posterior belly of the digastric muscle and trace the muscle upward and backward to the point where it dips beneath the mastoid process. At this stage, identify the main trunk of the facial nerve. Deepen the sulcus between the parotid gland on the one hand and the external meatus and mastoid process on the other so that the edge of the bony meatus can be identified.

7. At this stage, use the hemostat to splay out the bands in the sulcus and seek the facial nerve by blunt dissection. Insert a hemostat into the gland immediately superficial to the main trunk of the nerve and open it up in order to establish a plane. Insert a suitable retractor into the plane to retract the superficial lobe of the parotid forward and to allow identification of the bifurcation of the nerve. Slide the hemostat over the upper division and open the blades.

8. Incise the glandular tissue overlying the posterior blade using the Fugo blade upward and back-ward to divide the posterior border of the gland. Identify all branches of the facial nerve and divide the glandular tissue superficial to the nerve. (It is very easy to dissect this glandular tissue; it feels like you is cutting a piece of cake.) In this way, the superficial lobe is mobilized up to the upper border of the gland. Repeat the procedure to mobilize it from the zygomatic arch.

9. Then divide the lower half of the posterior and the inferior border using the same technique along the inferior division and consecutive branches.

Postoperatively not much seepage occurs in the drain-ing chamber wound. It heals nicely within 1 week. No complications have occurred during any of the sur-geries we have done.

Uvulopalatoplasty with Tonsillectomy

Uvulopalatoplasty is commonly used to alleviate snor-ing. Uvulopalatoplasty with tonsillectomy (Fig. 50.9) is used to treat snoring accompanied by mild obstructive sleep apnea.

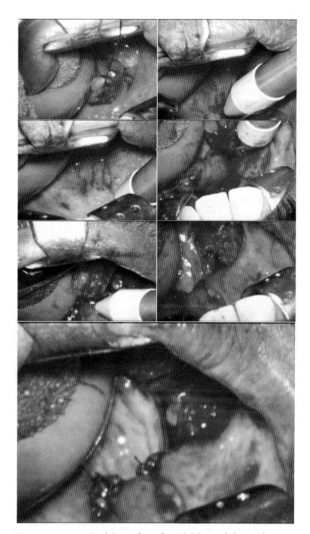

Figure 50.9. Excision of uvula. Division of the soft palate muscle along with tonsillectomy is done with the Fugo blade with no charring of tissue.

Reduced postoperative pain, fewer complications, and hence less morbidity and better compliance are some of the advantages of using the Fugo blade in this proce-dure. Postoperative hemorrhage and palatal insufficiency are lower; the patient heals more quickly as compared with conventional surgical methods. Finally, standard laser-assisted uvulopalatoplasty required multiple sittings to stiffen the palate and achieve the required results. The Fugo blade makes this a one-stage procedure.

Pharyngeal Stenosis

A 45-year-old woman was involved in motorcycle acci-dent in which she was partially strangled by the dupatta (a traditional scarf worn around the neck) she was wearing. She suffered injuries to the larynx, including fracture of the hyoid bone, thyroid cartilage, and cricoid cartilage and avulsion of the epiglottis. There was history of pain around the neck and immediate respiratory distress for which an emergency tracheostomy had been performed. The patient later presented with dysphagia, for which nasogastric feeding was started. Then the patient underwent pharyngeal dilation using a laser. Three attempts were made to relieve the stenosis, but each attempt led to further worsening of the condition. After this, the patient had to undergo a feeding jejunostomy. She was advised to undergo a total laryngectomy as well. The patient presented to me after this advice. The computed tomographic (CT) scan showed complete closure of the pharynx with a normal glottis. The supraglottic portion of the larynx was unidentifiable (Fig. 50.10).

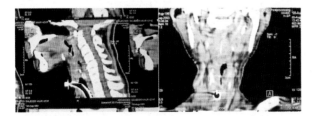

Figure 50.10. CT scans showing severe pharyngeal stenosis.

The patient underwent exploration of the neck with the Fugo blade and complete excision of the scar tissue (Fig. 50.11).

At present, the patient still has a minitracheostomy to maintain a normal airway. She has undergone decannulation repeatedly, but with little success because the jejunal graft, being a muscular tube, remains collapsed most of the time. She can swallow normally and has good, understandable speech. To speak, she must block the tracheostomy tube with her thumb. However, the patient is otherwise pursuing a normal life with no difficulty with regard to her respiratory, speech, and deglutitory functions.

We believe that the successful management and cure of this case is entirely due to the distinct advantages (better tissue definition, negligible thermal damage and scarring, better healing, less fibrosis) that the Fugo blade offers over conventional surgical methods and lasers.

The Ear, Nose, and Neck

Keloid on the Ear Lobule

The Fugo blade has proved to be an effective and easy instrument in the excision of keloids of the ear lobule (Fig 50.12) (and at other sites, including the chest wall

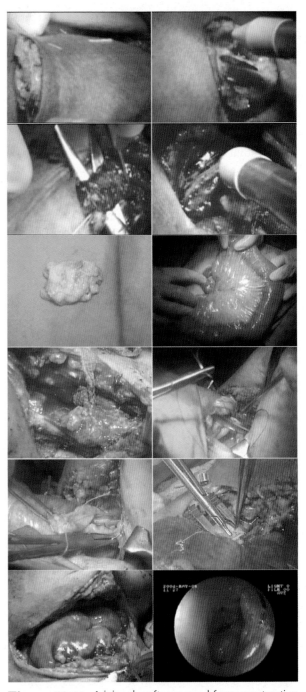

Figure 50.11. A jejunal graft was used for reconstruction of a muscular tube from the base of the tongue to the upper end of the esophagus and was also stitched to the soft tissue around the glottis.

and upper arm). Compared with conventional treatment methods, recurrence of keloids is negligible when treated with the Fugo blade. Several cases of recurring keloids were followed over a period of 3 years after surgery with a Fugo blade; not a single case showed evidence of recurrence.

We have also used the Fugo blade to excise a preauricular sinus.

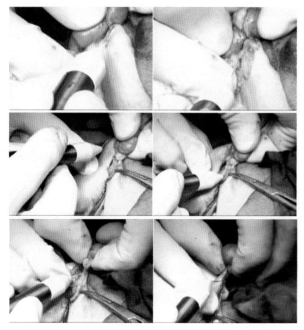

Figure 50.12. Steps of operation showing excision of a keloid using the Fugo blade.

Other Sites

I have successfully used the Fugo blade to treat septal papilloma and to excise nasolabial cysts, branchial cysts, and branchial sinus.

Summary

Although originally created for ophthalmic applications, the Fugo blade has proved to be an ideal substitute to enable ENT surgeons to provide patients with all the benefits of laser-assisted ENT surgery. Current applications of lasers can be damaging to the delicate vocal fold, especially in cases of juvenile laryngeal papillomas. The advent of the Fugo blade has led to better anatomical and physiologic results. It has definitely improved the quality of patient care.

Suggested Reading

Feder RJ. Laryngeal granuloma as a complication of CO2 laser. *Laryngoscope.* 93:944–945.

Myssiorek D, Persky M. Laser endoscopic treatment of laryngoceles and laryngeal cysts. *Otolaryngol Head Neck Surg.* 1989;100:538–541.

Ossoff RH, Werkhaven JA, Dere H. Soft-tissue complications of laser surgery for recurrent respiratory papillomatosis. *Laryngoscope.* 1991;101:1162–1166.

Rosen CA, Woodsen GE , Thompson JW, et al. Preliminary results of the use of indole-3-carbinol for recurrent respiratory papillomatosis. *Otolaryngol Head Neck Surg.* 1998; 118:810–815.

Shikowitz MJ, Abramson AL, Freeman K, et al. Efficacy of DHE photodynamic therapy for respiratory papillomatosis: immediate and long-term results. *Laryngoscope.* 1998; 108:962–967.

51 The Fugo Blade in Dermatology RAKESH BHARTI and DALJIT SINGH

Over the past four decades, the practice of dermatology has evolved from a subspecialty to a full-fledged specialty, and it is still evolving. Dermatosurgery is almost a superspecialty for most young dermatologists, who use cutting techniques and tools to gain ever better results.

Dermatosurgery is the branch of dermatology in which conditions refractory to medical treatment are dealt with and cosmetic improvement of the skin is thus brought about. Skin biopsies, excision of cysts and corns, ear lobe repairs, mole removal, and nail avulsion in cases of onychomycosis are all now being done by dermatosurgeons.

Common dermatosurgery procedures involve electrosurgery (which uses electrically generated heat), cryosurgery, or both (Tables 51.1 and 51.2). The Fugo blade can be of help in managing most of the conditions listed, as demonstrated by the following two case examples.

CASE STUDIES

Case 1: Tuberous Sclerosis

This 14-year-old patient had extensive nodule formation on the face. The diagnosis was tuberous sclerosis.

As a preliminary trial, the patient's right cheek was partially treated after the injection of local anesthetic. Two weeks later, the patient and his parents thought that the treatment substantially improved his face. There was no scarring and no inflammation. It was

Table 51.1. Common Electrosurgery Techniques

Electrofulguration	Small epidermal lesions such as verruga plana, milia, dermatitis papulosa nigra, and skin tags are removed by electrofulguration with a "fine epilation needle" electrode. In electrofulguration, superficial tissue is charred by sparks from the electrode, without actually touching the tissue.
Electrodesiccation	This involves touching the lesion with the electrode with a marginally higher current. Conditions such as seborrheic keratoses, verruca vulgaris, granuloma pyogenicum, cherry angiomas, and senile lentigines are removed by electrodesiccation followed by curettage.
Electro-epilation	This is a permanent hair-removal technique useful in hirsutism and cosmetic awareness for facial hair where the hair follicle is destroyed by various electrical techniques such as thermolysis, electrolysis or blend.

Table 51.2. Common Dermatologic Conditions Treatable with Cryosurgery

Benign	Warts
	Molluscum contagiosum
	Cystic acne
	Acne scars
	Keloids
	Granuloma pyogenicum
	Prurigo nodularis and mucoid cysts
	Xanthelasma and xanthomas
	Seborrheic warts
	Epidermal nevi
	Mucosal lichen planus
Premalignant	Leukoplakia
	Bowen's disease
	Actinic keratoses
Malignant	Basal-cell carcinoma
	Lentigo maligna
	Squamous-cell carcinoma <3 cm in size

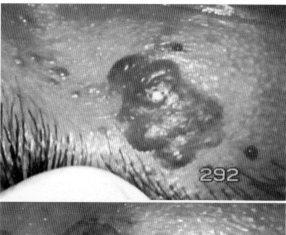
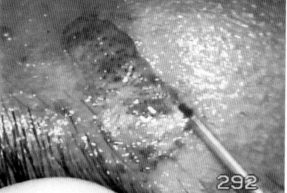

Figure 51.1. A large lesion is ablated from the edge inward.

then decided to treat the whole of the face under general anesthesia.

Surgical Technique

1. Use a 600-μm Fugo blade at medium power and high energy setting.

2. Depending on the size of the lesions treat them as follows. Touch small lesions and press vertically for a fraction of a second. This is enough to remove them.

3. For larger lesions, press the activated tip and rub it in a circular motion from the center outward until the area became flat. Rub the largest lesions from the top and the sides until the skin is flat. During ablation, if a large lesion becomes dry, the plasma energy has lost its effect, so periodically wet the lesion with saline. In our case, it took over an hour to treat a few hundred lesions on the face (Fig. 51.1).

In our case, removing the lesions from all parts of the face was easy, but it was especially so on the nose and nasolabial folds, where there was firm tissue underneath.

Postoperative Management

Seven days after surgery, our patient's face was relatively clear. He was vastly better than before and was in high spirits (Figs. 51.2 and 51.3).

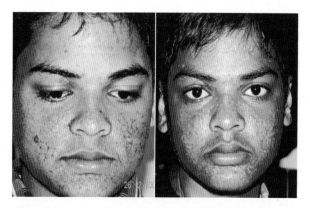

Figure 51.2. A part of the right cheek had already been treated with the Fugo blade as a trial. The rest of the face was treated in one sitting. **Left:** The patient 7 days after treatment. **Right:** Seven days after treatment left cheek.

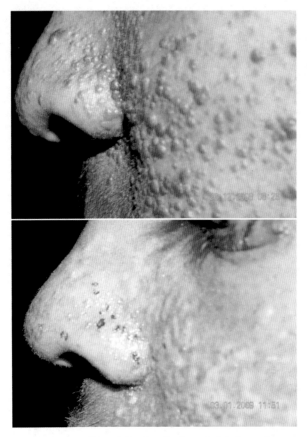

Figure 51.3. Part of the face before and 7 days after Fugo blade ablation.

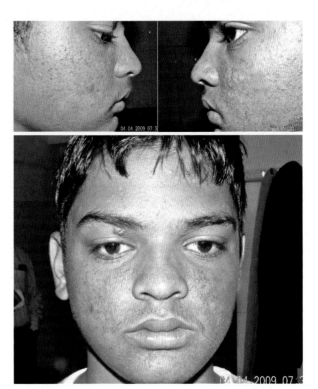

Figure 51.4. The patient 1 month after Fugo blade ablation. The number and size of the lesions are greatly reduced.

One month later, the condition had improved further. The uneven pigmentation over the face had lessened. However, hundreds of small lesions remained that merited further surgical attention. One large lesion on the right upper eyelid and several lesions on both cheeks had not shrunk and these, too, required additional treatment (Fig. 51.4).

Once again, under general anesthesia, the patient's entire face was "touched up" as in the previous surgery. Figure 51.5 shows the patient 2 week after subsequent surgery. If the patient wishes greater skin smoothness, additional sessions can be scheduled. But the Fugo blade will not cause burning and scarring, as is common with current classic dermatologic surgical tools.

Case 2: Palmar Corn

The patient was a 65-year-old woman with a large corn on the palm of her hand. The corn was in a prominent position on the palm and caused pain when it was banged or bumped. Under the care of a dermatologist, she had received three intralesional injections of steroid over a 6-month period, but the corn did not resolve. The Fugo plasma blade was used to surgically remove the corn.

Lignocaine was injected under and around the lesion. The front of the lesion was sliced with a 100-μm Fugo blade tip and the deeper layers and the walls were removed with a 600-μm Fugo blade tip. The 600-μm tip removed the tissue more slowly and simultaneously stopped any bleeding. Finally, the base and sides were cleaned up a 300-μm tip. The dissection was clean, and no clinically visible damage to healthy tissues occurred. The raw edges were brought together with superficial 80-μm steel sutures (Fig. 51.6). Recovery was uneventful and the sutures fell off after 12 days (Fig. 51.7). One month after surgery the skin at the surgical site appeared normal (Fig. 51.8).

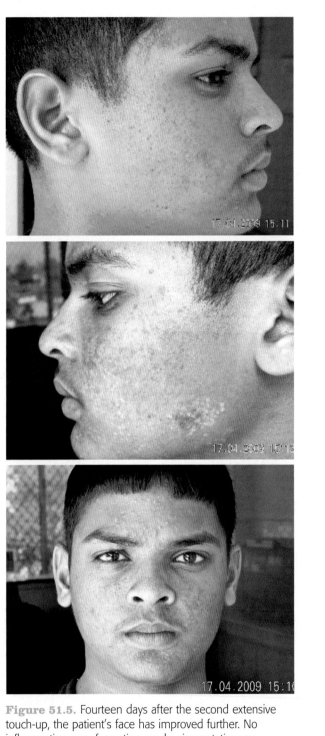

Figure 51.5. Fourteen days after the second extensive touch-up, the patient's face has improved further. No inflammation, scar formation, or dyspigmentation are present.

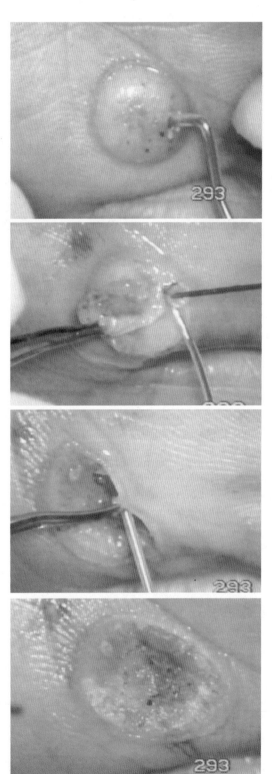

Figure 51.6. A first attempt to remove the corn was made with a 600-μm Fugo blade tip, to see how it would react to ablative energy from a thick tip, but the result was unsatisfactory. The lesion was then sliced with a 100-μm Fugo blade tip. The side walls were cleared with 600-and 300-μm tips.

51

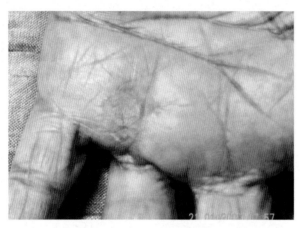

Figure 51.7. Twelve days after surgery, the operated area still appears rough.

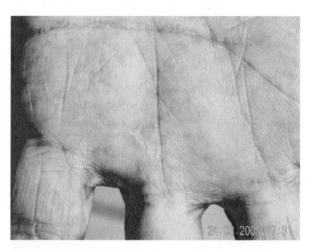

Figure 51.8. One month after surgery, the skin appears near normal.

Summary

If a difficult condition like tuberous sclerosis can be successfully treated with a simple ablative tool like the Fugo blade, then it is likely that many common and rare skin conditions can be treated with no risk of inflammation or scarring.

The two cases described above were a challenge to the current armamentarium of dermatosurgeons. The Fugo blade, however, easily corrected these conditions. It appears that dermatosurgery will undergo a revolution with the use of the Fugo blade.

Suggested Reading

Darke DB, Morgan RF, Cooper PH. Shave excision and dermabrasion for facial angiofibroma in tuberous sclerosis. *Ann Plast Surg.* 1992;28:377–380.

Dvir E, Hirshowitz B. The use of cryosurgery in treating the fibrous papules of tuberous sclerosis. *Ann Plast Surg.* 1980;4:158–160.

El-Musa KA, Shehadi RS, Shehadi S. Extensive facial adenoma sebaceum: successful treatment with mechanical dermabrasion: case report. *Br J Plast Surg.* 2005;58:1143–1147.

Fischer K, Blain B, Zhang F, et al. Treatment of facial angiofibromas of tuberous sclerosis by shave excision and dermabrasion in a dark-skinned patient. *Ann Plast Surg.* 2001;46:332–335.

Hori K, Soejima K, Nozaki M, et al. Treatment of facial angiofibroma of tuberous sclerosis using cultured epithelial autografts. *Ann Plast Surg.* 2006;57:415–417.

Janniger CK, Glodberg DJ. Angiofibromas in tuberous sclerosis: comparison of treatment by carbon dioxide and argon laser. *J Dermatol Surg Oncol.* 1990;16:317–320.

Pantelis A, Bootz F, Kühnel T. Laser skin resurfacing and fibrin sealing as successful treatment for facial angiofibromas in tuberous sclerosis. *HNO.* 2007;55:1009–1011.

Pasyk KA, Argenta LC. Argon laser surgery of skin lesions in tuberous sclerosis. *Ann Plast Surg.* 1988;20:426–433.

Swaroop MR, Nischal KC, Rajesh Gowda CM, et al. Radiofrequency ablation of adenoma sebaceum. *J Cutan Aesthet Surg.* 2008;1:89–91.

Afterword

The Future of the Fugo Blade

Richard J. Fugo, M.D., Ph.D.

A senior executive of a large ophthalmic company once commented that the Fugo blade is the first paradigm shift in the art of tissue incision since the introduction of the laser in the mid-1900s. I agree. To date, the world has used the Fugo blade micro-ablation system in ophthalmology and dentistry with four U.S. FDA clearances while operating from flashlight batteries. Now, a novel micro–macro Fugo ablation system is in use that operates from batteries or plugs into wall current. The system offers a fiber-optic attachment that provides imaging in high definition. This system is still portable and offers the real possibility of revolutionizing most fields of surgery. As an example, the system offers the hope of eliminating at least 50% of open heart surgeries. This novel system has the possibility of resistance-free incision through a 2-mm perforation site that leaves pristine clean incision walls, kills any microbe on contact, provides prolonged antimicrobial properties to the incision, causes hemostasis without incision-wall cautery, and allows the surgeon to weld the incision wall closed rapidly and safely. In conclusion, this is a technology that will be used by the entire world fraternity of physicians to improve the level of health care worldwide.

Appendix

Literature References to the Fugo Blade

A chronological listing of the Fugo blade in the medical literature.

1. Sabbagh LB. The never-ending quest: creating a better way to remove the lens. *Eyeworld*. 1998;3:50–53.
2. Sabbagh LB. The leading edge: harnessing electrons for a faster, smarter incision. *Eyeworld*. 1998;3:88.
3. Kronemyer B. Fugo blade uses low-level energy to create anterior capsulotomy. *Ocular Surg News*. 2000;18(21):45–46.
4. Kellan R, Fugo RJ. Device increases safety, efficiency of cataract surgery. *Ophthalmol Times*. 2000;25:7–9.
5. Fugo RJ, DelCampo DM. The Fugo blade™: the next step after capsulorrhexis. *Ann Ophthalmol*. 2001;33:12–20.
6. Singh IR, Singh D, Singh R, et al. The plasma blade in vitreoretinal surgery. *Ann Ophthalmol*. 2001;33:280–289.
7. Samalonis LB. Improving capsulotomies. *Eyeworld*. 2001;6:42–44.
8. Winn CW. Broad applications seen for electrosurgical instrument. *Ocular Surg News*. 2001;19(11):45–46.
9. Roy FH. Course for Fugo blade is enlightening, surgeon says. *Ocular Surg News*. 2001;19:35–38.
10. Winn MC. Broad applications seen for plasma blade. *Ocular Surg News/Asia-Pacific Edition*. 2001;12(8):1–5.
11. Kent C. Plasma capsulotomy. *Ophthalmol Manage*. 2001; 5:72–73.
12. Singh SK. Fugo blade capsulotomy: a new high tech cutting technology. *Trop Ophthalmol*. 2001;1:14–16.
13. Singh IR. Vitreo-retinal surgery with plasma blade: a case report. Trop Ophthalmol. 2001;1:13–16.
14. Singh IR. Managing proliferative vitreo-retinopathy with the Fugo blade—a case report. *Trop Ophthalmol*. 2001;1:24–25.
15. Singh D. Singh micro-filtration for glaucoma: a new technique. *Trop Ophthalmol*. 2001;1:7–11.
16. Fugo RJ. "PhacoXcap" using the Fugo blade. *Ocular Surg News*. 2002;20:12.
17. Kent C. PhacoXcap: a new procedure makes it possible to phaco both nucleus & cortex outside the capsular bag. *Ophthalmol Manage*. 2002;6:80.
18. Kent C. Revealed: the eye's lymphatic system. *Ophthalmol Manage*. 2002;6:114.
19. Fugo RJ. The plasma blade: taking cataract surgery to a new level. *Ophthalmol Manage*. 1999;3:51–54.
20. Singh D. Use of the Fugo blade in complicated cases. *J Cataract Refract Surg*. 2002;28:573–574.
21. Singh IR, Singh D, Singh R, et al. Vitreoretinal surgery with plasma knife may be a new frontier. *Ocular Surg News*. 2001;19:80–83.
22. Fine IH. Fine on phaco. *Eurotimes*. 2002;7:1–5.
23. Fine IH, Hoffman RS, Packer M. Highlights of the 2002 ASCRS Symposium, Part I. *Eyeworld*. 2002;7:38.
24. Bethke WC. A new clue to lymphatic drainage? *Rev Ophthalmol*. 2002;9:12.
25. Bethke WC. Is PhacoXcap right for you? *Rev Ophthalmol*. 2002;9:37.
26. Fugo RJ. PhacoXcap cataract surgery. *Ann Ophthalmol*. 2002;34:12–14.
27. Singh D. Peep-hole surgery for dacryocystitis. *Trop Ophthalmol*. 2002;2:11–12.
28. Kent C. Transciliary filtration—without bleeding. *Ophthalmol Manage*. 2002;6:84–87.
29. Hoffman RS. New dimensions in cataract surgery. *Ophthalmol Manage*. 2003;Buyer's Guide:45–48.
30. Singh D, Singh K. Transciliary filtration using the Fugo Blade. *Ann Ophthalmol*. 2002;34:183–187.
31. Hidalgo-Simon A. Plasma knife provides clean and accurate cut for capsulorrhexis. *Eurotimes*. 2002;7:27
32. Fugo RJ, Singh D, Fine IH. Automated Fugo blade capsulotomy: a new technique and a new instrument. *Eyeworld*. 2002;7:49–54.
33. Charters L. Cataract surgeons gain better control with capsulotomy blade. *Ophthalmol Times*. 2003;28:16.
34. Video journal of cataract and refractive surgery. *New Developments New Devices Fugo Blade*. 2002;18(1).
35. Singh D. Conjunctival lymphatic system. *J Cataract Refract Surg*. 2003;29:632–633.
36. Singh D, Singh RSJ, Kaur H, et al. Plasma powered squint surgery with the Fugo blade. *Ann Ophthalmol*. 2003;35: 12–14.
37. Singh D. Pediatric cataract: my experiences. *Trop Ophthalmol*. 2002;2:7–12.
38. Fugo R. Regarding transciliary filtration. *Trop Ophthalmol*. 2002;2:7–8.
39. Singh D. Transciliary filtration & lymphatics of conjunctiva—a tale of discovery. *Trop Ophthalmol*. 2002;2:9–13.
40. Kent C. Capsule rims: an issue of strength. *Ophthalmol Manage*. 2003;7:61.
41. Eisenstein P. World's smallest knives. *Popular Mechanics*. 2003;180:56–58.
42. Ronge L. How to use the Fugo blade. *EyeNet*. 2003;7:23–24.
43. Wunder H. Why be an ophthalmologist-inventor? *Rev Ophthalmol*. 2003;10(9):25.
44. Young M. Fugo blade finds its niche in difficult cases. *Eyeworld*. 2003;8:70.
45. Fugo R. The Fugo blade allows new surgical maneuvers. *Ocular Surg News*. 2003;21:5–7.
46. Guttman C. Study supports safety for Fugo blade capsulotomy. *EuroTimes*. 2004;9:20.
47. Guttman C. Anterior capsulotomy benefits from new technology. *Ophthalmol Times*. 2004;29:16–17.
48. Singh D, Singh RSJ, Singh K, et al. The conjunctival lymphatic system. *Ann Ophthalmol*. 2003;35:99–104.
49. Fugo R. The Fugo blade: practice and patient benefits. *Admin Eyecare*. 2004;13:87–90.
50. Kent C. Minimizing zonular stress with the plasma blade. *Ophthalmol Manage*. 2004;8:157.
51. Wolf K. Surgeon describes learning curve with Fugo blade. *Ocular Surg News*. 2004;22:10.
52. Kent C. FDA approves new glaucoma filtration procedure. *Rev Ophthalmol*. 2004;11:6–8.
53. Izak AM, Werner L, Pandey SK, Apple DJ, Izak MGJ. Analysis of the capsule edge after Fugo plasma blade capsulotomy, continuous curvilinear capsulorrhexis, and can-opener capsulotomy. *J Cataract Refract Surg*. 2004;30: 2606–2611.
54. Guttman C. Anterior segment tool proves ideal for many applications. *Ophthalmol Times*. 2005;30:14,16.
55. Guttman C. Transciliary filtration provides improved safety and simplicity. *Ophthalmol Times*. 2005;30:28.
56. Fugo R. Transciliary filtration procedure offers new approach to glaucoma. *Ocular Surg News*. 2005;23:4–26.
57. Fugo R. Cushioned PhacoXcap technique addresses difficulties with small pupils, hard cataracts. *Ocular Surg News*. 2005;23(7):16–17.
58. Singh D, Singh RSJ. Applications of the Fugo blade. In: Wilson ME Jr, Trivedi RH, Pandey SK, eds. *Pediatric cataract surgery; techniques, complications, and management*. Philadelphia, Pa: Lippincott, Williams & Wilkins, 2005:97–100.

59. Scimeca G. Phaco with transciliary filtration an alternative to triple procedure. *Ocular Surg News*. 2005;23:58.

60. Fugo R. Transciliary filtration procedure offers new approach to glaucoma. *Ocular Surg News*. 2005;16(6):18–19.

61. Fugo R. A new way to perform trabeculectomy. *Ophthalmol Manage*. 2005;8(1):53–54.

62. Atwal A. "Atwal's balanced approach" for glaucoma filtration surgery presented. *Ocular Surg News*. 2005;19:64–66.

63. Kent C. Corneal pits may relieve edema. *Rev Ophthalmol*. 2005;9:6–8.

64. Peponis V, Rosenberg P, Reddy SV, et al. The use of the Fugo blade in corneal surgery: a preliminary animal study. *Cornea*. 2006;2:206–208.

65. Wilson ME, Trivedi RH. Technological advances make pediatric cataract surgery safer and faster. *Tech Ophthalmol*. 2003;1:53–61.

66. Wilson ME. Anterior lens capsule management in pediatric cataract surgery. *Trans Am Ophthalmol Soc*. 2004;102: 391–422.

67. Fugo RJ. Mature cataracts: how to breeze through them. *Ocular Surg News*. 2006;24:8–9.

68. Peponis V, Rosenberg P, Reddy SV, et al. Study finds Fugo blade can be of use in corneal surgery. *Rev Ophthalmol*. 2006;8:94.

69. Singh D. Fugo blade used to clear cloudy corneas. *Ocular Surg News*. 2006;24:54–58.

70. Wilson MR. US case reports add to experience with corneal ablation pits. *Ocular Surg News*. 2006;24:56.

71. Trivedi RH, Wilson ME Jr, Bartholomew LR. Extensibility and scanning electron microscopy evaluation of 5 pediatric anterior capsulotomy techniques in a porcine model. *J Cataract Refract Surg*. 2006;32:1206–1213.

72. EyeWorld Staff. Relatively new surgical tool has multiple uses. *Eyeworld AP Today*. 2006;August 14:4.

73. Fugo RJ. Fugo blade to enlarge phimotic capsulorrhexis. *J Cataract Refract Surg*. 2006;32:1900.

74. Fugo RJ. Strategy for capsulotomy. *Cataract Refract Surg Today*. 2007;7:15.

75. Fugo RJ. Fugo blade capsulotomy. *EyeNet*. 2007; July/August:11.

76. Singh D, Kaur A, Singh K, et al. Sutureless levator plication by conjunctival route: a new technique. *Ann Ophthalmol*. 2006;38:285–292.

77. Singh D. Orbicularis plication for ptosis. *Ann Ophthalmol*. 2006;28:185–193.

78. Singh D, Bundela R, Agarwal A, et al. Goniotomy ab interno: "a glaucoma filtering surgery" using the Fugo plasma blade. *Ann Ophthalmol*. 2006;38:213–217.

79. Fugo RJ. Trans-ciliary filtration. *Video Journal of Current Glaucoma Practices*. 2007;1(2).

80. McGrath D. Fugo blade effective tool for multiple surgical applications. *Eurotimes*. 2008;13(6):43.

Index

Page numbers followed by *f* and *t* indicates figures and tables, respectively.